Amazing Days, Endless Nights

Mystique of Surgery Three

by
David Gelber

The narrative is based on real patients and events; however, names and details have been altered to protect individual privacy.

To Contact the Author:
www.davidgelber.com
david@ruffianpress.com

ISBN-13: 978-0-9820763-8-5
ISBN-10: 0-9820763-8-X

First Edition – 2018

Typesetting/Interior Layout Design by Giánna Carini
http://www.giannacarini.com

Cover Design by Elizabeth Little
Hyliian Design
https://www.deviantart.com/hyliian

Caduceus Cover Vector © http://123rf.com/abdulrohim

Amazing Days, Endless Nights

Mystique of Surgery Three

by
David Gelber

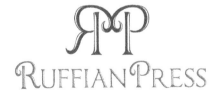

RUFFIAN PRESS

DEDICATION

To all my patients.

INTRODUCTION

Previously I've taken you *Behind the Mask* and *Under the Drapes*, two books which provided a glimpse into the wonders of the operating room, unveiling the mystique of surgery. Now it is time for new journeys, extraordinary cases, memorable hours and days, complicated surgeries, patients who kept me standing in the operating room for hours, made me work through the night, sometimes for days, all in the effort to mend broken and diseased bodies and souls.

The stories are roughly chronological, starting with medical school, moving on to residency, and finally out into the world of private practice where I've toiled for more than twenty-five years.

Names and details have been changed or altered for privacy. The injuries, diseases and operations all actually occurred. Each chapter tells a story of the most amazing days and many endless nights which were spent saving lives and stamping out disease.

MEDICAL SCHOOL MOMENTS

The first year of medical school was a jumble of lectures and labs punctuated with brief encounters with actual live patients.

My first clinical encounter was a half day at one of the local Emergency Rooms where I was joined by a fourth-year student. I'd been in med school for about three weeks. These weeks had allowed me to become well versed in the anatomy of the back muscles and the histology of the liver and spleen, but I knew nothing of authentic diseases or their treatment.

We met one of the ER attendings, an internist, and I was treated to a few hours of medical hieroglyphics. We were quizzed on the therapy for urinary tract infections, a pretty simple question. As I began to answer, the fourth year spouted off a litany of different antibiotic choices, drowning out my suggestion of Penicillin. At that time in my medical career I thought Penicillin was *the* antibiotic and was effective treatment for any and all infections. This may have been true in 1945. But, it was now 1980 and the list of antibiotics was growing longer every day. I stayed quiet for the final few hours, listening and learning rather than demonstrating my ignorance.

My next encounter with real patients was a four-week elective in Urology, myself along with two of my classmates. Our instructor was Dr. Leake. We also had two sessions with Dr. Cockett. Leake and Cockett. Can you think of two more appropriate names for Urologists? One of the highlights of these four weeks was visiting Mr. Godfrey.

Unfortunate Mr. Godfrey had cancer of the prostate and was in the hospital receiving combined radiation and hormonal therapy. We saw him twice a week, and as part of each visit, Dr. Leake wanted us to do a rectal exam on poor Mr. Godfrey. This twice weekly torture was supposed to allow us to appreciate the progress of Mr. Godfrey's therapy. Without even a sigh, Mr. Godfrey turned on his side and suffered through this biweekly ritual. The last session of this elective finally came which meant the last four rectal exams Mr. Godfrey would have to endure. We all arrived sporting those big "We're Number One" gloves frequently seen at sporting events.

"OK, Mr. Godfrey, time for your rectal exams," we chimed in unison.

Dr. Leake was not amused, but our patient had a nice chuckle.

There were no other memorable clinical encounters until the third year. The entire class eagerly began "General Clerkship." Four weeks were allotted to teach us how to talk to, listen to, and touch the, up until now, sacred, hallowed creature called, "The Patient."

We were told to let the patient talk, to listen actively and guide the patient down the history road so that they would impart as much information as possible. We were taught how to guide a rambling patient back to the clinical path which would then lead to the formulation of the all-important "Differential Diagnosis." Thus, it was emphasized over and over, the history would guide the next steps of a patient's evaluation.

We discussed the philosophical and practical concerns along with the grave responsibility that accompanied the "Laying On Of Hands." The actual physical exam meant we were given permission to burst through societal taboos against penetrating another individual's personal space, sometimes invading their most personal and intimate parts, always, we were told, towards the goal of healing.

"Just the act of physical touching may be beneficial to your patient's wellbeing," one psychiatrist lectured.

We were treated to Dr. L demonstrating a complete physical exam (except rectal and pelvic) on one of our classmates. He spent about forty-five minutes observing, palpating and auscultating, in the end declaring: "As you can see, this complete physical need not be an all-day affair."

In our more modern times, when a primary care physician may see 50-60 patients a day, performing a forty-five minute exam on each patient would make for a very long day indeed.

We all waited with fear and trepidation for the "Pelvic Day." This was the day when each student would receive indoctrination into the intricacies of the female pelvic exam. Professional models were hired, each set up in a private cubicle where the student was given about ten minutes of monitored groping... I mean probing.

"My uterus is retroflexed," my model reported, "so you would need to do a rectal exam to properly feel it. You should be able to feel each ovary, however."

"Until you've done about two hundred pelvic exams, you may as well be waving your fingers in the wind," Dr. A, one of our instructors, commented.

Finally, the last pieces of the physical exam came up: the aforementioned rectal exam and the male genital exam. These we did on each other. "Never go to a Proctologist who can palm a basketball," one instructor joked.

"You should be concerned if you feel both your examiners hands on your shoulders during a rectal exam," another quipped.

"All in good fun to lighten the tension," they said. Maybe they should have volunteered to be subjects... all in the name of education, of course.

Finally, we were finished with general clerkship and were ready to be set loose upon the unsuspecting patients of Rochester, New York.

"Go do an H&P on the new admission in 612, a Gertie Black, CHF," my third-year resident ordered.

Ready or not here I come, Ms. Black.

I perused the chart of patient Black before venturing in to see her. I glanced across the nurse's station into her room and caught a glimpse of my new patient. She was about five feet tall and five feet wide. At the precise moment I looked over at her, she bent over. Her hospital gown did little to cover her ample assets and I was treated to a "full moon over Rochester." So went my introduction to clinical medicine at Strong Memorial Hospital in Rochester, New York.

It wasn't long before I was churning out handwritten 10- to 15-page H&P's on a daily basis. The history part, the H, was not a problem. Ask the right question and listen. My patients had no qualms about opening up to me, revealing the darkest secrets of their lives.

"I... like... to smoke... a few... joints... every day... well... several... times... a day," Mr. M. confided. He had been doing this for most of his seventy years. His very measured, deliberate speech no longer was a surprise.

"I prefer women's underwear," another man confided. "It's more comfortable."

"I put my cat in the drying machine when I was seven," an elderly woman reported. I really didn't think it was relevant to her having hemorrhoids, but one never knows.

"I drink a little every day, maybe three beers a day, and a couple of glasses of wine, and I have two martinis after dinner and a brandy at bedtime, but, I'm not an alcoholic," a councilman confessed.

And so it went.

The intricacies of the physical exam, the P, were more of a challenge.

As a class we shared our interesting heart murmurs, palpable lumps and bumps, hernias, rales, rhonchi, and wheezes. Gradually, I thought I was developing some physical exam proficiency.

Then came my day. I was chosen to present to Dr. M on rounds. My patient was Cora, sixty years old, with COPD and Congestive Heart Failure, admitted with shortness of breath.

I questioned her every way I could, going back to her childhood days, looking for any every possible contributing factor to her severe COPD. I tried to anticipate any and all questions.

I examined her from top to bottom and then bottom to top. She had a barrel chest, an S3, mild JVD, expiratory wheezing and, I decided, a right ventricular heave.

I wasn't really sure about the right ventricular heave, whose definition follows:

When there is pulmonary hypertension, the right ventricle has to overwork, it has to pump against the increased pressure in the lungs. So if the heel of the hand is placed immediately lateral to the LEFT sternal border, one can feel the right ventricle being pushed anteriorly. The heel of the hand is lifted off the chest wall with each systole, and this is the heave.

I'm still not sure if I felt anything. But, I read it was associated with severe COPD and poor Cora certainly qualified. I convinced myself it was present. And, this was my chance to impress the attending staff.

My moment came.

"Cora is a sixty-year-old female who was admitted to the hospital complaining of shortness of breath...two packs of cigarettes a day for forty years...distant breath sounds bilaterally...right ventricular heave...being evaluated for lung transplant."

Silence.

I've done it. They're speechless. I'm sure they've never been so dazzled by a med student.

"Dr. Gelber," Dr. M began, "could you demonstrate how one examines a patient and determines the presence of a right ventricular heave?"

Wait, I know this.

"Good morning, again, Cora," I greeted her as I moved to her bedside. "I need to check your chest."

"Whatever you need to do, Dr. G." She turned to Dr. M. "Dr. G's a good doctor. He spent an hour with me yesterday, just listening and checking me. It's OK, go ahead and do what needs to be done."

I put my hand alongside her sternum. Unfortunately, I put it on the right side and felt nothing.

"I'm not sure it's there," I murmured softly.

"It would probably help if you put your hand in the proper spot," Dr. M. observed.

"Oh, yeah," I stammered, even more softly.

I moved my hand to the proper spot and still felt nothing.

Dr. M. moved in. he put his hand along the left sternal border, watched her breathing, and then turned to our group.

"Definitely no right ventricular heave," he announced. "Maybe, Dr. Gelber, you should be a surgeon."

A seed was sown.

TYING KNOTS

L ast week in surgery one of the surgical techs commented on how fast I could tie knots. I was a bit surprised, to tell the truth, because I've never considered
myself a "fast" surgeon. During my training I was always impressed by those surgeons who were technical
wizards, whose fingers could dance across a patient's
insides and dissect quickly, cleanly, and precisely. I had
always thought of myself as more of a plodder, working
methodically towards a defined goal, doing my best to
stay out of trouble while trying to accomplish the task
at hand.

I try to have a plan for every operation I perform,
simple or complex, and then find the safest way to reach
the end, attempting to anticipate each potential pitfall
and sidestep them as much as possible. I usually say,
"I'm not a slow surgeon, I'm not a fast surgeon; I'm a
half-fast surgeon."

But what of the knot-tying comment. The first thing
any medical student learns about the technical aspects
of surgery is how to tie knots. During my medical school
days, if one wanted to do anything in surgery besides
become close friends with the end of a retractor, one had
to demonstrate the ability to tie surgical knots.

This skill always began with a friendly surgical intern, at least one friendly enough to take pity on a help-

less ignorant medical student. Such an intern would demonstrate and instruct the proper way to tie knots. First, two-handed tying, and then the cooler one-handed techniques. The student would then procure several yards of suture and spend the night tying knots to armchairs, tables, dogs, cats, fellow students, and anything else that was handy.

Armed with this newly perfected skill, the student would enter surgery the following morning poised to demonstrate this newly honed talent. Of course, before the eager med student would get his or her chance, it was necessary for the operation to be done. The tedious bowel resection would drag on and on until the attending or Chief resident would announce to the second-year resident that it was time to close. If the Chief resident left the OR, the second-year would hand the suture to the intern who would then close the abdomen.

The first layer closed would be the fascia, the most important layer. The fascia is the layer with the most strength and its closure would always be under the watchful eye of a senior resident; third-year medical students never were allowed to close this layer. But, next would come the subcutaneous tissue, a layer that added no strength to the closure; a layer composed mostly of fat which could be sutured or not. There is some theoretical benefit to closing this layer, eliminating so-called dead space, but it mostly allowed interns some practice in suturing.

So the intern sutures this layer closed and then, the big moment, asks the medical student to tie the knot. The student carefully pulls on each end of the suture and throws the first knot; so far so good. The second knot is thrown and it settles about a centimeter from the tissue, leaving a big gap and the suture doing nothing, the first knot having loosened up while the second knot was being tied. The student then tries to cover up this error in technique by cinching down on the suture, hoping it will slide down to its proper resting place. Instead the suture breaks and the intern is forced to start over, muttering something about the suture breaking due to the "jerk" at the end of the string.

But, after this initial false start, the medical student is given a second chance. For some reason, living tissue is very different from the arms of chairs. This time the student ties the knot and holds tension as the second knot is thrown and manages to get it cinched down to the tissue, only this time the extra tension causes the suture to tear completely out of the flimsy fat, leaving our hapless student holding a suture with two perfectly tied knots, but holding nothing but air together.

At this point most interns would instruct the student to practice a bit more while finishing the work themselves. Most medical students, having been thoroughly humiliated, would try to spend the remainder of their surgical rotation reading *Schwartz* while planning a future in dermatology. The exceptional, intrepid student, however, perseveres. If said student is extremely bold he will ask for one more chance. Given this opportunity, the student then ties three perfect knots, the tissue stays together properly, and this student spends the rest of the day with a smile on his face, having taken the first small step that leads to a life surrounded by gowns, masks, gloves, blood, guts, worry, success, failure, life, and death.

A future surgeon is born.

FIRSTS

Our lives are full of firsts.

Parents wait for their baby's first tooth, first words, and first steps.

We may remember our first day of school, first solo bicycle ride without training wheels, first automobile drive, first date, first kiss, first sexual encounter, and other firsts that I can't recall at the moment.

A surgeon also has firsts.

I clearly recall the first surgery I ever saw. Now, you might think that because I am the son of a surgeon that my childhood was replete with trips to the hospital with my father where I accompanied him into the OR and became his right hand man at the age of thirteen.

Not true.

On rare occasions I did go to the hospital with my father. He would go to make daily rounds, but the closest I ever got to an operating room was sitting on a bench outside the gift shop, watched over by the volunteer behind the cash register while my father went upstairs to see his patients.

Far more lively and interesting were the occasional conversations at the dinner table which delved into the world of surgery.

Dad: "Dr. A, the anesthesiologist, is getting a divorce. Isn't his wife, Betty, in your Bridge Club?"

Mom: "She's the reason the bottle of Scotch is almost empty."

Dad: "Well, she was sleeping with Dr. K while Dr. A went off and spent a weekend with one of the nurses in the OR."

Mom: "I guess I'll need to find somebody new for the Bridge Club, one who doesn't like Scotch. Anything new at work?"

Dad: "My new office nurse is pregnant."

Mom: "You mean the one who said she hadn't been able to get pregnant for two years? She's only been with you for two months."

Dad: "I guess some of the Gelber fertility rubbed off on her,"

Mom: "That's the third nurse who's gotten pregnant in the last eighteen months. And, none of them had been able to get pregnant before."

Dad: "It must be something in the air."

Back to the topic, there have been many important medical "firsts" over the years. I remember my first day of medical school. I met Herman, my anatomy group's cadaver who was to be a constant companion through the first semester, and I met Sigrid, last name Gelber, my lab partner. She quickly became my adopted sister and friend through medical school and afterwards. She had survived osteogenic sarcoma at age seventeen and had suffered through initial rejection of her med school application because no one thought she would survive long enough to finish out the four years of school. She did finish, married, and was a highly regarded specialist in Pediatric Endocrinology at Northwestern University until her untimely death from breast cancer at the far too young age of 35.

Then there was my first day of internship, a Sunday. I arrived at the hospital where I was greeted by a list of patients and instructions from my second-year resident to make rounds, do the necessary H&P's on the new admissions, and he would see me the next day. I couldn't even find the bathroom, let alone a myriad of patients. This particular resident, not surprisingly, was fired before the year was out and is now tormenting surgeons as an anesthesiologist.

It was as a first-year medical student that I actually witnessed my first operation. I was assigned an advisor, Dr. C. Nelson, a Neurosurgeon. His job was to smooth the transition from the rigors of college to the even greater exactitudes of medical school. I don't remember much of what he did as advisor, except that he invited me to watch an operation. He was performing a trans-sphenoidal resection of a pituitary tumor the following day. Finally, something more than the formaldehyde of anatomy and squinting into a microscope in Histology.

I managed to find my way to the OR, assisted by an OR nurse who directed me to the locker room where I donned the blue surgical scrubs of Strong Memorial Hospital, 60% Cotton, 39% Polyester and 1% stainless steel.

After several wrong turns, I stumbled into OR room six where the operation was about to commence. I managed to come within six inches of contaminating the scrub tech's back table, while I looked upon the patient, prepped and draped with her upper lip pulled back, exposing her teeth and gums.

"This patient has Nelson's Syndrome caused by a tumor in her pituitary gland," Dr. Nelson explained.

"We'll approach the pituitary through her sphenoid sinus, which is behind her maxilla."

I nodded my head, then asked, "Is Nelson's Syndrome named after you?"

"I wish," he answered. "That was a different Dr. Nelson."

I watched as the Chief Resident began the surgery, incising above the teeth, removing bone, and finally reaching the pituitary gland. An operating microscope was wheeled into position and Dr. Nelson began the real operation. I was able to watch through a second teaching port.

I saw some reddish tan stuff and then some yellow gray gunk, and then I saw Dr. Nelson tease the yellow gray gunk away from the reddish tan stuff.

"The thin grayish tissue is the adenoma. She's making too much ACTH which is causing her adrenal glands to secrete too much cortisol, resulting in her having Cushing's disease."

"I thought you said she has Nelson's Syndrome?" I asked in my ignorance.

"Nelson's Syndrome is causing her to have Cushing's disease," he explained, displaying far more patience than I deserved.

After a few hours the operation was finished. The Chief Resident closed her up, sealing the surgical site with some fat and superglue.

"It looks painful," I commented as he glued the bone back in place, while I considered what it would feel like to have someone cut me along my upper gums.

"Surprisingly not," the Chief Resident responded.

"How do you learn to do such an operation," I wondered out loud.

"I take notes, read about the technique, assist on cases, and then do the surgery," he answered. "It's all about studying and observing."

One thing he didn't mention was innate talent. When I finally began doing surgery I realized that technical skill was something that could be taught only to a certain extent, natural ability played a bigger role. Truly great surgical technicians are born, not made, at least in my opinion.

It was years after this first experience with surgery that I actually performed my first real surgery. It was my first month of internship and I was on call when Peter was admitted to the "resident's" service. He'd had abdominal pain for three days, with nausea, vomiting, and elevated White Blood Cell count. He had exquisite tenderness in the right lower quadrant of his abdomen. Peter was a textbook case of acute appendicitis.

It was about 7:00 pm when my Chief Resident, Dr. S, and his attending, Dr. T., joined me in the OR for Peter's appendectomy. I had read the book on appendicitis and studied the technique over and over.

The surgical tech handed me the scalpel and I began to make my incision.

"You're shaking like a goddam Parkinsonian," commented Dr. T.

I did shake a little, but not enough to interfere with the actual surgery.

Once the incision was made, I switched to the electrocautery and buzzed the bleeders in the skin edge and then made the incision deeper until I saw the diagonal fibers of the external oblique fascia. Just like in the book, I incised in the direction of the fibers and retracted this muscle.

"Take a Kelly clamp and split the muscle of the next layer along the direction of their fibers. First with the muscle, then perpendicular to it so that it spreads apart. By the way, which muscle is this?" Dr. S asked.

"Internal Oblique," I answered without losing a beat.

"Right. If you didn't know, then I would have to take over the surgery," he added.

The Internal Oblique and Transversalis muscle fibers were split apart exposing the peritoneum.

"Clamp," I requested.

The scrub tech slapped it into my hands, just like in the movies.

I picked up the peritoncum with the clamp.

"Another clamp for my assistant," I said, a bit too softly.

"What?"

"Another clamp for my assistant," I replied, much more loudly.

"OK, OK, you don't have to yell," the tech added.

I opened the peritoneum and some cloudy fluid poured out.

"Culture," I said loudly and I was handed a swab.

"Now, put your finger in and see if you can feel the appendix," Dr. S instructed.

"I feel something hard," I replied.

"Let me check," he suggested as he put his fingers through the opening in the peritoneum. "That should be the worm (nickname for the vermiform appendix, the complete name for the appendix); see if you can flip it up into the wound."

I put my finger in and swept it around the offending organ and it came into view. It was swollen to the size of a Hebrew National Knockwurst.

"Don't grab the appendix," Dr. T. barked. "Find the cecum."

Years later another attending surgeon, Dr. Bronsther, taught me this one surgical nugget about appendectomies; it was the only thing I ever learned from him.

"Appendectomies are surgery of the cecum."

What he meant was that the appendix always arises from the cecum, which is the first part of the colon. It is always found where the three tenia coli, which are the three longitudinal muscle layers which are seen on the colon, coalesce. Over the many years I've been doing appendectomies, these two pearls of wisdom have served me well.

Back to Peter. I identified the cecum, gabbed it with a Babcock clamp, and delivered it up into the wound. Once enough of it was protruding through the wound, I grabbed it with a sponge, rocked in back and forth until the entire cecum popped into the wound, followed by the very swollen and inflamed appendix.

Now it was time to actually do the surgery, that is, remove the sick organ.

"Wait, wait," Dr. S. said forcefully.

The three of us stared at the swollen appendix, greatly enlarged all the way to its base. The normal procedure would be to divide the mesoappendix, which carries the appendiceal artery, ligating the blood vessels, then divide and ligate the appendix close to the cecum, usually leaving a small stump. There was controversy in those days about inverting the stump or merely tying it. The consensus was that simple double ligation was appropriate. Inverting the stump potentially created future problems.

"Start with the mesoappendix?" I wondered out loud.

"Right," Dr. S. agreed.

We clamped along the fat which led to Peter's appendix and then tied each blood vessel within the clamp until the appendix was free from any attachments all the way to the cecum. There was a short segment, about three millimeters, of normal appendix.

"Clamp it there?" I suggested, pointing to the uninflamed stump.

"Yeah, but use a Kelly on the appendix side," he added.

Clamp, clamp, cut, and that sick appendix was gone.

"O Vicryl tie?" I requested, a touch of doubt in my voice.

"Right," my assistant agreed, "and we'll need some 2-0 Vicryl stick ties, also."

We tied off the appendiceal stump and then sutured the cecum over this ligature. I admired my handiwork for a moment.

"Put it back where it belongs, Dr. Halsted," Dr. S. ordered. "The patient's not getting any younger."

I closed him up, irrigating and suturing each layer before stapling the skin closed. Peter was wheeled off to Recovery as I trailed slightly behind holding his chart and sporting a big grin on my face. He went on to an uneventful recovery.

Years later, during an interview, I was asked about my most memorable moments. I cited two:

My wedding day and Peter's operation.

24

Back in the day, that is the distant past of 1985, the word "internship" often filled a medical student with anxiety and stress. The internship was a rite of passage, a necessary stop on the road to becoming a full-fledged, finished doctor, rather than a person with a couple of initials after his or her name.

And, the Surgical Internship was supposed to be the worst: 36-hour shifts, every other night call, holding retractors for hours without a break, this was the plight of those of us who chose to pursue the surgical arts. It was a period of initiation which led to joining an exclusive fraternity called "Surgeon."

I have to report that, at least for me, my internship was nothing like this. I was in a large private hospital where there was no "scut" work, the name given such mundane tasks like drawing blood, starting IV's, doing EKG's and such. These duties are important to patient care, but do little to advance the knowledge of the medical trainee. I do think there is some value in learning to draw blood and start IV's, but doing my own CBC's or urinalysis would have been a waste of my time.

All this being said there were days when the work was never ending and there is one day in particular which stands out as a shining example of what an internship can be.

It was during my final month, a month I spent away from the safe confines of my mother hospital and its friendly IV, EKG, and phlebotomy teams; thus the aforementioned "scut" work still plagued the lowly intern. I finished out my intern year rotating through the Pediatric Surgical Service at Children's Medical Center (CMC) in Dallas. This included responsibility not only for CMC, but also Parkland Hospital, the county hospital for Dallas. I was paired with a fourth-year resident as well as interns and residents from the program at UT Southwestern. We were responsible for all the pediatric surgery which included elective surgeries, trauma, the Parkland Emergency room, surgical consultation for pediatric patients in both hospitals and, finally, the nascent Pediatric Liver Transplant program.

The intern's duties included: history and physical on all admissions, morning rounds which commenced around 6:00 a.m., drawing blood on all the liver transplant patients, which was to be done *before* morning rounds, assisting in surgery, afternoon rounds, making sure all tests that had been ordered had been done and being the first to respond to any emergency that should arise throughout the day. In between all this we all hoped to find the time to actually do some surgery, the occasional appendectomy or a hernia, remove some lumps and bumps, and so on.

There was a day, an unforgettable day, which snuck up on me about two thirds of the way through the month. It was a Saturday which started like every other day. I arrived early enough to help the intern coming off call draw blood on the liver transplant patients and to check on my other patients before the fourth-year resident arrived and formal rounds began. So far, so good.

Round and round we went, from Children's Medical Center, to Parkland, which included a brief stop in
the newly minted, but as yet untested, Pediatric Trauma
Unit. There was a post op appendectomy, the previously mentioned post liver transplant patients, including
little Terry. Terry had received her new liver four days
ago, but was still looking green. We were all concerned
that something wasn't right. Diagnosing and treating
her was priority number one for this Saturday.

"See if Radiology can do an ultrasound of Terry's
abdomen with Doppler to check her hepatic artery," the
transplant surgeon attending commanded.

"Yes sir," the fourth-year resident agreed.

Rounds ended and this fourth-year resident, who
aspired to be a Pediatric Transplant Surgeon, which
meant an unusual amount of groveling and brown nos-
ing of the attending staff, turned to me and gave me the
job of tending to all of Terry's needs.

It was 7:00 a.m. and the proverbial shit was poised
to hit the fan. I started at the top of the scut list and ran
down to Radiology to request the stat ultrasound on
Terry. I checked the requisition up and down and front
to back, made sure all the t's were crossed and i's were
dotted, and ventured in to find the senior radiology resident. I finally found him hidden away in a dark corner,
which is the usual place to find radiologists, the vam-
pires of the medical world who shun all light and live
in shadow. I begged and pleaded and convinced him of
the urgent need. I have to admit I almost brought tears
to his eyes as I related the "Plight of Baby Terry." The
ultrasound was scheduled stat.

One task settled, I moved on to the daily mundane
chores an intern battled. In those days, before comput-
ers, I gathered lab results and X-Ray reports and started

writing my progress notes on each patient. It wasn't too long when I received the first of many "rude" interruptions.

"Dr. Gelber," a sweet voice called, "we've got a premie down here in NICU with a distended abdomen and the KUB shows pneumatosis."

A bothersome but occasionally disastrous NEC watch. One more thing to complicate what was turning out to be a far from peaceful Saturday.

What, pray tell, is "NEC" watch?

NEC stands for Necrotizing Enterocolitis. This is a condition which most commonly arises in premature babies. Whether from ischemia or infection or some other unknown agent, the bowel becomes inflamed and the neonate becomes very sick. The child cannot be fed, they demonstrate signs of sepsis and their condition can deteriorate before your eyes.

I made my way to the NICU and took a look at baby girl Nicole born at 28 weeks and now sporting all the findings one would expect in early NEC, distended abdomen, mild tachycardia, and an abdominal X-Ray which revealed an area of "pneumatosis intestinale" which means *air in the wall of the bowel*. I communicated my findings and assessment to my fourth-year resident, specifically that baby Nicole should be watched, tube feedings were put on hold, and she was to start on IV fluids and antibiotics.

One crisis stopped before it started, I hoped.

I had just hung up the phone with the senior resident when my beeper went off.

Parkland ER. Just great, what now?

"You are the surgery intern on call today?" asked the voice from the ER.

"This is Dr. Gelber; I am on call today."

"This is Dr. Barry. We've got a seven-year-old who we think has appendicitis. Do you think you can come check him out?"

"OK, I'll be there in a little bit."

I took the time to write a couple of progress notes on the patients I'd seen earlier in the day and then made my way through the tunnel which connected Children's Medical Center and Parkland. It was like moving from one world to another.

CMC always looked new and clean. It was a place I would want to bring my kids if they were ill. Parkland, although not dirty, looked older and worn, a place which looked beaten down by years of caring for the sickest, most severely injured patients Dallas could offer.

I found Mikey in the pediatric ER accompanied by his worried mother. He had been sick for three days. From the doorway it was obvious he was ill. He lay still on the exam table, his face was flushed. The bedside chart listed Vital signs: Heartrate 130, Temp 103.1, Blood Pressure 86/40, Respirations: 20.

A typical history for appendicitis was obtained and a gentle tap on his abdomen elicited a grimace and wincing that screamed "PERITONITIS."

I called my senior resident again and scheduled Mikey for surgery. My beeper went off again: *Call the transplant floor.*

"Terry needs to go for abdominal ultrasound now. The radiologist is here and you need to bring her," the unit secretary informed me.

Four years of college, four years of medical school, and almost a year of internship, and I'm still just a glorified orderly.

"OK, I'll be right up."

I left orders for Mikey and called the OR and told them I would call when we were ready for surgery. One good thing about Mikey and most patients with appendicitis was that an appendectomy was an intern case, so I would get to do the operation. I hustled my way back to CMC to wheel little Terry to ultrasound. On my way my beeper went off again and again and again.

"Michelle has a temp of 102."

"Michelle who?" I inquire.

"Michelle S. in 204, She had a liver transplant ten days ago."

"Oh, that Michelle. Get a UA, draw two sets of blood cultures and a CBC. I'll be over to check her shortly."

"Are you going to come draw the blood?"

"Yeah, OK, I'll get to it as soon as I can."

Next.

"IV is out on Darren in 331."

"Darren?"

"He had an appendectomy two days ago."

"Is he eating?"

"Clear liquid diet."

"Is he on any meds?"

"Ampicillin, Gentamicin, and Clindamycin."

"Any fever?"

"No fever for twenty four hours."

"Was the appendix ruptured?"

"How should I know?"

I looked at my sign out sheet. No mention of how bad the appendix was.

"OK," I finally answered. "Could you please put everything at the bedside and I'll be there when I can."

And the third call:

"Dr. Gelber, Scott in 320 has a headache…"

Finally, something simple.

Now, onto the Transplant floor and little Terry. She was very small for her age and her skin was green because of her liver failure. Even after her transplant she stayed green and now she had fever. Everything said her new liver wasn't right. But, the question remained: Was it a technical problem? Or rejection? Or infection? Thus the ultrasound and Doppler of her hepatic artery which would start to provide some answers, we hoped.

The nurses already had her loaded up on the stretcher. We began wheeling her down the hall to the elevator. She gave me a weak smile. Father and Mother trailed behind us talking in whispers. Terry was four days post-transplant. I knew her fairly well and was very well acquainted with the veins of her right arm where I drew her blood every morning. Her mother was only worried, while her father seemed to mix his worry with distrust, as if the Transplant team was somehow conspiring to harm his little girl.

The radiologist and the transplant attending were waiting for us. The ultrasound clearly demonstrated a patent hepatic artery and we brought Terry back to her room. On the way my beeper went off again. It was my Chief resident. It was a good time to do the appendectomy on Mikey. I called the OR and met the team in the ER and we wheeled our patient up to surgery.

With my Chief across the table from me, I started the surgery. This was the final month of my internship and I was pretty adept at appendectomies. I delivered the offending organ, which was ruptured, and completed the surgery like a pro. Mikey had just settled into the recovery room when my beeper went off again. Terry was crashing.

I raced through the tunnel and up the stairs to her bedside. My Chief was right behind. Her nurse wasted no time informing me that an ICU bed was ready. Terry was barely responsive, her BP was 50/0 and she looked even greener. I scooped her up in my arms while her father stood behind me screaming.

"If she doesn't get better, you'll never work in this city again," he shouted. I think he would have punched me if he had the chance.

Meanwhile I laid her in the ICU bed. The pediatric anesthesiologist was standing by and deftly intubated her while the nurses opened up her IV and gave her a bolus of fluid.

"Rejection," the transplant attending decided.

Terry was now functioning without a liver, more or less; her transplanted liver was causing more harm than help. She was placed at the top of the list so that the first ABO compatible liver that came available would be hers. Her father came in and stood at her bedside, glaring at me while I stood at the foot of the bed staring at the monitors. Her BP was better at 70/40 and her oxygen saturation was 100%. Still, she wouldn't last long without a new liver.

It was early evening now and I finally had a few moments to catch up. I finished my charting for the day, drew some overdue blood tests, and started a few IV's which had been waiting for me. I was about to have "breakfast" when my Chief called me.

"A two-year-old girl is on her way by helicopter to the Trauma ICU. She was accidentally run over by her father."

A minute later the call came. I was already on my way.

A crowd of nurses and paramedics surrounded the stretcher as Christina was wheeled inside.

"BP 60/30, Heart Rate 125, O2 Sat 100%," a nurse screamed.

Two clear but terrified eyes stared up at me as my Chief arrived just behind me. Christina was awake and alert and breathing comfortably. She watched intently with her beautiful blue eyes; eyes which displayed trust but also terror. A quick survey revealed bruising across her lower abdomen and pelvis and blood staining her diaper, coming from her perineum. There was obvious deformity of both legs.

Two distraught parents waited outside as the trauma team went to work. New IV lines were established and fluids administered. Blood was drawn for the blood bank and baseline lab tests. Antibiotics were given, oxygen administered. We did a quick peritoneal tap which was negative. Her vital signs were holding steady.

X-rays revealed a fractured pelvis and bilateral femur fractures. Her chest X-Ray was normal.

The OR was standing by and at 8:57 p.m. surgery commenced. My job, as intern, was holding retractors as the attending and Chief resident began the task of putting her lacerated perineum back together. Her vagina was torn down the middle and there was a small laceration of her rectum. Her fractures were to be treated without surgery, at least at this time.

The surgery dragged on, past nine o'clock, past ten o'clock, past eleven o'clock. All the while messages came: Baby A needs a new IV, Mikey has a fever, Terry's urine output is low, and on and on. As midnight approached I began to see bright spots before my eyes. The OR lights started to spin as tiny beads of sweat appeared on my forehead. My heart began to pound against my sternum, trying to jump out of my chest.

I can't remember. Have I eaten anything today? I don't think so. Let's see: light headed, tachycardia, diaphoretic...

"Do you think you can find me some orange juice or something?" I asked the circulator. "I haven't had much to eat or drink all day and I'll bet my blood sugar is approaching zero."

The nurse must have felt sorry for me and managed to find some apple juice and fixed it up with a straw which allowed me to suck it down in a few seconds. A few minutes later I was back among the living as the sugar filled my bloodstream. I was able to continue my relationship with the end of a Richardson retractor without passing out. Finally, shortly after one-in-the-morning, the vaginal and perineal repairs were finished. All that was left was to do a colostomy. I begged to be allowed to leave and finish all my undone work and to check on my other sick patients.

My superiors took pity on me and I was dismissed. I scrounged up a couple of Oreo cookies and went about the business of catching up. I checked on Terry first, gave her some more fluid and was informed that there was a potential liver in Houston. I started IV's, answered calls for patients with fever or drainage from their wounds, drew the morning labs, and thought I could see a glimmer of light at the end of the tunnel.

Christina was now back in the Trauma ICU and she looked stable, if not a little forlorn as she lay in bed with both legs up in traction, IV's in each arm, and tubes going every which way. However, she was OK and she still had those beautiful clear blue eyes, only now I didn't see the terror.

Then my beeper went off. It was the ICU where Terry was clinging to life.

My Chief answered: "There's a compatible liver in Houston. We're leaving in ten minutes. Make rounds with the next crew and then you can go. We won't be starting the surgery until about ten.

And there it was. My twenty-four-hour shift was now growing to twenty six. I did take a few minutes to get a real breakfast before starting morning rounds with the next team of residents.

Rounds were uneventful. We finished around 8:30, but instead of leaving to get a little rest, I stayed around to help with Terry. Dedication or stupidity? Both, I guess, but I assume it was mostly dedication and a sense of responsibility.

We started Terry's surgery at around 10:30 and I took my position on the patient's left where I would become reacquainted with my old friend, Richardson. The case went fairly quickly, at least for a liver transplant and after about two hours the new liver was in place. Everyone left to take a break, that is, everyone but me. Someone had to stay with the patient, who was still under anesthesia while the new liver "breathed." I sat and watched the liver take on new life as Terry's blood percolated through its sinusoids and it started to sweat bile. After about thirty minutes the rest of the team returned to do the final step, which was the biliary anastamosis.

I was happy to see the intern on call for that day return with them, which meant I was to be set free. It was almost two in the afternoon. My twenty-four-hour shift had lasted thirty two; a typical day for a surgery intern in 1985.

Christina, by the way, made a complete recovery. Mikey spent about a week in the hospital but also recovered, while Nicole recovered from her NEC. Terry's new liver worked for a few days, but she suffered through another rejection, and this time it was too much and she passed away.

Modern medicine does indeed have its limitations.

FOURTH OF JULY

I was now a newly minted second-year resident and it was the Fourth of July, my second night taking call at the county hospital.

I am ready for anything, I thought.

"Call ER, Dr. Gelber."

It was 9:15 a.m.

"We've got a fifty-year-old male with a stab wound to the abdomen," the ER attending reported.

And so it started.

I made my way down there and found Jose. He was stable and there was a two cm wound just above his umbilicus.

In those days we usually locally explored the wound, and if it penetrated the peritoneum, the patient was taken to surgery.

I called for some local anesthetic, an instrument tray, and some retractors. Just as I had learned as an intern, I extended the stab wound and followed it down, down, down, deeper into the abdominal wall. Through fat, more fat, then fascia, then muscle, then more fascia I explored. After five minutes I found peritoneum and the stab wound kept going.

Looks like he's going to the OR.

We, that is myself and my interns, got him typed and crossed, started antibiotics, and called my Chief, a fourth-year resident.

"I've got Jose here with a stab wound to the abdomen, penetrates the peritoneum. I think he needs to go to surgery. He's stable and he should be ready whenever you are."

Twenty minutes later, off he went.

Maybe I can finish some of the work I need to do. Write some progress notes, check some X-Rays.

"Beep...beep...beep."

ER again?

"Twenty-nine-year-old male with a gunshot to the chest and abdomen just rolled through the door."

"I'm on my way," I answered. I then started my fast walk back down to the ER. Sometime during medical school I decided that there are very few emergencies that require me to run. If the patient is so sick that I have to be there ten seconds sooner, then he probably wasn't going to survive, no matter what I did. But, I can walk pretty fast.

Miguel was rolling into Room 4 as I arrived. He was awake with a BP of 90/50, heart rate of 110.

"Do you have any medical problems?" I asked. "Any allergies to medicine? Do you take any medicine regularly? Any surgery for anything in the past? Can you tell me what happened?"

"I was sittin' on my porch reading the Good Book when these two dudes came up and shot me, 'Bam, Bam,' " he explained. "I wasn't doin' nuthin'."

"What about any other medical history?" I asked again.

"No, I never go to the doctor, ain't never been sick, don't take no meds or drugs. Don't drink o' smoke," he answered.

"Ok," I sighed. "Let's get another IV going, and get him a gram of Mefoxin."

I gave him the once over. He had one wound in his right chest which exited his right lower back and a second wound in his lower abdomen which went straight through. Tattoo's extolling the virtue of his mother and his love for Angie adorned his chest and back. A large scar ran from his left shoulder to his mid forearm.

"What's this scar from?" I wondered out loud.

"Cut myself shavin'," he answered and then he smiled.

"Type and Cross for four units PRBC's. Let's get a single shot IVP to make sure he's got kidneys, and I'll need a chest tube tray, and he'll need a chest X-Ray," I barked out, hoping either the nurse or my intern was paying attention.

I called up my Chief again.

"Gunshot wound to the chest and abdomen for you," I reported. "I'm about to put in a chest tube and then we'll take the picture for the IVP. He'll be headed your way in about thirty minutes or so."

And so it went.

Andrew came in with a stab wound to the right chest, the result of him losing an argument over a girl.

He earned a right chest tube and entered the queue to go to surgery.

Next came Miriam, complaining of severe abdominal pain. She said it started after she had rough sex with her boyfriend.

"How rough," I asked as politely as I could.

"Well, I was laying on the bed like this…" she spread her arms and legs, "…and Billy, that's my boyfriend's name, was at the foot of the bed and he jumped on top of me. I got the wind knocked out and then my belly started hurting really bad."

"Did Billy come with you?"

"I'm right over here, Doc," a voice called from the doorway.

There was Billy, about six-foot-three, at least three hundred pounds.

"Is that what happened?" I asked.

"Just like she said," he replied.

I palpated her abdomen. She was diffusely tender, more in the left upper abdomen. I looked at the monitor: heart rate 130, BP 100/60.

I turned to the nurse.

"Give her a liter of LR and send blood for type and cross, and I need a peritoneal lavage tray."

The nurse pointed to the cabinet, intimating that I should help myself to the tray.

I walked my intern through the procedure. As she slipped in the lavage catheter, bright red blood shot out.

"I'd call that positive," I observed and we pulled the catheter out.

I called my Chief again and Miriam was whisked away to the OR.

I had just made it up to the ICU to check on some of our other post-op patients when my beeper went off. The number for the ER popped up.

Will it never end?

John arrived, hypotensive, complaining of severe abdominal pain. He'd stayed drunk for most of the last three weeks and now he had all the findings of severe pancreatitis. He was admitted to the ICU, required intubation and ventilator support, and was dead six days later. Over the course of his illness he exhibited ten of Ranson's eleven criteria for predicting mortality from severe pancreatitis. Six or more and mortality is predicted to be 100%.

It was four in the afternoon now and I sensed a lull in the stream of sick and injured. The day wasn't half over and I'd already done a week's work.

My Chief called and asked me to come up to the OR where they were about to wheel Miriam in to Room 4 for her surgery.

"Dr. M is taking a break. Come and do this case with me, that is, if the ER has settled down."

"Seems quiet at the moment. I'll be there in a minute."

Performing surgery is always the best part of being a surgeon. I hustled over to the OR and we spent the next hour and a half taking out Miriam's spleen. At surgery it looked like the spleen had exploded, leaving bits and pieces held together by clotted blood.

I hope Billy let's her go cowgirl for a while.

No sooner had I tucked Miriam away in the recovery room when my now despised beeper went off and the familiar number to the ER appeared.

"Five MVA's? Give me a break," I cried, but then headed down to the ER, my home for most of the next twelve hours.

They were waiting for me, five patients strapped to back boards, faces splattered with blood and bits of glass. Their car had driven off a bridge and plunged about fifteen feet into a ravine.

"Chest X-Ray, Femur X-Ray, Pelvis X-Ray, CT of head, C-Spine X-Ray, start another IV, Type and cross-match. Let's go, let's go!"

And so we went, nurses and my two interns sat with the patients as they made their way from the ER to X-Ray to the CT Scanner, and then back to the ER.

Fractured femurs, fractured tib fib, fractured pelvis, right pneumothorax, left pneumothorax, tension pneumothorax, multiple rib fractures all made an appearance in one of those patients.

"Call Ortho. Call Neurosurgery. Call Urology."

And with all the injuries, none of those five needed a general surgery procedure outside of a chest tube.

No sooner had I finished shipping the last of the MVA's off to ICU when Eli came in by ambulance, gunshot wound to the head. He was breathing, but very shallow, heart rate was 100 and BP was 100/60. There was dried blood on the right posterior scalp and the defect in the skull was palpable. He did not move the left side of his body.

He was intubated with the help of a friendly nurse anesthetist and was taken away for CT of his head, one of my interns babysitting. There was a brief lull amid the chaos which allowed me to accompany them. I kept a close eye on Eli and my intern.

The CT revealed extensive injury to the right posterior brain with bits of bone and bullet mixed in.

I called the Neurosurgeon on call and then prepared Eli to go to OR where he was to have the wounds debrided and ventriculostomy inserted. It was now 8:06 p.m. and the admission count stood at eleven. The night was still young.

Eight thirty came and went without another call, but eight thirty three brought two more stab wounds, one with multiple abdominal wounds and the other with one to the chest and each arm.

Back to the routine: "Tell me what happened? Do you have any medical problems? Any surgery in the past, any allergies, do you smoke? Drink? Use drugs? Take any medications?"

The abdominal wound was easy to assess as a big wad of omentum was hanging out of the abdominal wall. Antibiotics, type and cross, and off to the OR.

The second one had a hemopneumothorax and superficial wounds to the arms. A right chest tube delivered 800cc blood and then nothing more. The patient was stable, the post chest tube X-Ray looked good and, with any luck, he would not need any further intervention. He was trundled off to the intermediate care unit. ICU beds were becoming precious. Two more bad patients and I would need to go begging for beds in the Medical or Cardiac ICU's.

As if on cue, the ER called again. This time it was Barbara, fifty years old, with right lower quadrant abdominal pain, nausea, vomiting, elevated white blood count. Everything to suggest acute appendicitis. I called Sara, one of the new interns, to go and evaluate her with the promise that she could do the surgery if Barbara truly seemed to have appendicitis.

Just as Sara ran off, the ER called again, gunshot wound to the leg was coming in. George, the other intern, and I arrived in the ER just as Maurice was being wheeled into one of the trauma rooms. He was awake and screaming. There was a big gauze bandage soaked in blood wrapped around his leg. I started my usual banter and he just screamed, the scent of alcohol permeated the room.

"Let me look at your leg," I requested with a bit of force in my voice.

"Get the fuck away from me," he answered.

"How about your foot?" I asked.

"Fuck off."

I took that as a yes and looked at his foot which was cold, blue, and almost lifeless.

"Maurice, I am sorry to tell you that you need to have surgery. It looks like the bullet has injured you femoral artery. If you don't have surgery you will almost surely lose your leg," I informed my belligerent patient.

"Fuck you."

"Does that mean 'fuck you, I want surgery' or 'fuck you, I'd rather lose my leg," I asked him.

He calmed down for a bit and agreed to surgery, and allowed me to finish my survey of him and his injuries. A few minutes later, he was up in surgery.

My pager went off again, only this time it was the OR calling. Sara was ready in the OR with Barbara and her appendicitis. I was to assist her, as the Chief was tied up with our stream of trauma patients. I was happy for a respite from the ER, which had reached a brief lull. I made sure no one was waiting that might need surgery and that there were no injured parties on the way, and then I made my way to OR 5.

It was 10:15.

Barbara's surgery took about an hour as I walked Sara through the appendectomy. She did a fair job. Of course my reprieve from the ER couldn't last. I had barely put my head down for a break when the call of the ER came again.

Another stab wound to the abdomen.

Back to the ER where I found Drew, nineteen years old, BP 70/40, heart rate 140, conscious, but barely.

"Need to intubate him and start another IV," I commanded, going into captain of the ship mode.

The nurse anesthetist easily slid the endotracheal tube in, we ran in a couple of liters of Ringer's Lactate IV fluid and he perked up a little. Blood pressure came up to 90/60 and heart rate fell to 120.

Poor Drew had a two-inch wound in the mid abdomen just above the umbilicus with a small amount of blood pooling. He was pale and thin and palpation in the wound went all the way in the peritoneal cavity, almost through to his back.

Blood was hung and I put the call into the Chief.

"This patient needs to go right away. He arrived hypotensive and we've got blood hanging now," I reported.

"Just finished one, three still are waiting, but they're stable. We'll come get him now. Keep up the good work," he answered.

A nice little pat on the head. It's two a.m., the bars are just closing.

Why do people feel the need to assert their manhood when drunk? Closing time until about three a.m. is prime time for the knife and gun club. Drunk and disorderly takes on new meaning as the nightly revelers leave the safe confines of the pub and saloon and wander into the street. Knives, fists, clubs, and guns raise their menacing heads.

"Hey, it's the Fourth of July... no, it's now the Fifth of July... people have been partying all day and night. I don't think there will be many more," I lied to myself out loud.

Like clockwork the ER called again.

"Two drunk guys with stab wounds, one in the neck, the other in the abdomen. Both look pretty stable."

I arrived in the ER just in time to see the ambulance wheel in a young boy, five years old, complaining of severe abdominal pain after being assaulted by his mother's boyfriend, thrown against the bathroom sink.

Devon looked up at me with sad brown eyes and winced if I even lightly tapped his abdomen. He was otherwise stable, although a little tachycardic with heart rate 120.

I also quickly evaluated my two stabbing victims, who, it turned out, had stabbed each other over the matter of twenty dollars and a pool match. The first was a stab to the mid neck which had penetrated through the platysmal layer and would best be treated with exploration. The abdominal stabbing also penetrated fairly deeply and would also need to go the OR.

I talked with the Chief again, who came to evaluate the child. As I was talking with him, my intern put up the boy's chest X-ray which revealed free intraperitoneal air.

"One more for the OR," I stated. My Chief just sighed.

"How many is that?" I wondered out loud. We'd both lost count.

Over the next few hours, three more MVA's arrived, all with a variety of fractures: ribs, femurs, humerus, tibias, fibulas, but nothing that would need general surgery. I performed the mundane task of admitting them and they were taken away to await their orthopedic procedures. It was time to make morning rounds.

It was six a.m.

With my two interns in tow, we started in the ICU, visiting the myriad pre- and post-op patients whom we had met in the twenty four hours we'd been on call.

As we finished, my Chief called.

"Dr. M is tired and he's leaving. We've got three more patients to explore. The stab wound to the neck, and two stab wounds to the abdomen. Come on over to the OR so we can knock these out.

So after spending almost an entire day in the ER, I finished up in the OR exploring a neck which had only a lacerated anterior jugular vein and a tiny tear in the thyroid cartilage, then doing exploratory laparotomies on two patients where I repaired six holes in the small bowel, resected a short segment of colon, and did a colostomy.

We checked on a few of the sicker patients before we left.

It was 3:25 in the afternoon.

By my count I had admitted twenty five patients, mostly seriously ill and injured.

Jose had suffered injury to his liver, colon, and mesenteric artery.

Miguel had been shot in the colon, stomach, and pancreas.

Miriam had shattered her spleen after her three-hundred-pound boyfriend had jumped on her spread eagled, naked body.

Maurice had suffered injury to his right femoral artery and vein. His leg was saved, but he remained obnoxious.

Eli survived his surgery, but succumbed to his massive head trauma forty eight hours later.

Drew survived injury to his diaphragm, stomach, spleen, and left kidney, walking out of the hospital after a two-week stay.

Devon suffered a perforation of the third part of his duodenum and a laceration of his pancreas. Timely surgery allowed the injuries to be repaired and he recovered uneventfully. His mother's boyfriend went to prison for five years.

Happy Fourth of July!!

MOOSE

His name belied his appearance. Moose should be a hulking, muscular middle linebacker with a voice which boomed across the room. He was short and thin, sporting thick glasses, but he introduced himself as "Moose."

"I can't swallow," he told us, succinctly summing up his problem in three words.

Indeed, he carried a towel with him which he frequently spit in, collecting the saliva which had no place to go.

Moose was short for Moose------r, his last name. His first name was Francis, but he had been called Moose ever since he could remember.

"I used to be bigger, that is heavier, but I've lost a lot of weight over the last year, about seventy pounds," he added after some prodding.

His story was classic for esophageal obstruction: progressive dysphagia, first for solids, then liquids, reaching the point where nothing, not even his own spit, would pass. Upper endoscopy by the GI service confirmed that Moose had carcinoma of the esophagus. Surgery would be needed, perhaps there was a chance for cure, but certainly an operation would palliate his miserable symptoms.

I was a fourth-year resident when I saw Moose. My Chief resident, Dr. J and *the* Chief, Dr. Di, our Chief of Surgery, were nearby and I presented Moose's case. The Chief loved esophageal surgery and cleared his schedule so that he could be present for Moose's operation. The plan was for a total esophagectomy via a combined thoracic and abdominal approach.

Pre-op workup was pretty much completed. The tumor was mid esophagus, appeared to be separate from all the vital mediastinal structures such as major bronchi and carina and major blood vessels, and there was no evidence of metastatic disease.

Moose was admitted to the hospital. He was five foot seven, 105 pounds. He had been a heavy drinker many years in the past, but had been sober for three years. He still smoked cigarettes. Otherwise he was in pretty good shape. Pulmonary function tests were performed which he passed with ease.

Surgery was set for Thursday, two days later.

"You think I'll be OK, Doc?" Moose asked.

"Don't worry," I answered, "we'll take good care of you and, when the surgery is done, you'll be able to eat a pizza sideways."

He smiled.

"Ah, to eat anything solid, that would be a treat," he remarked and then he stared up at the ceiling.

He added, "I don't know why I didn't see a doctor sooner. Something's been wrong for months. I knew it; I just didn't want to face the truth. Truth is I was scared, still am. But you have made me feel better."

"Well, it's not me doing the surgery. I'll just be helping Dr. Di and the Chief resident, Dr. J. I will be there for the entire surgery and I promise we will take good care of you afterwards."

I put my hand on his shoulder and then I left.

Moose rolled into OR 12 at 7:20 on Thursday morning. Anesthesia was induced without a hitch, appropriate monitoring lines were placed, and he was positioned on his back, but with his right side raised up to provide better access to his right chest.

At 8:12 Dr. J. made his abdominal incision. Dr. Di wasn't there yet, trusting Dr. J and me to do the proper exploration and mobilization of stomach. Dr. J was moving very slowly, even for him.

"Dr. Di is not going to be happy if he gets here and all you've done is free the omentum from the colon," I remarked.

"I need to be sure I do this right," he responded and went back to work.

I watched him plod along, a millimeter at a time and was tempted to pick up the tissue and scream: "Cut right along here," but I held my tongue and did my best to assist Dr. J.

As a resident, this sense of frustration was something I would experience over and over, never really getting used to it. I would be assisting another resident, senior, or junior, watching and sometimes cringing as they dissected or attempted to dissect, sometimes causing inordinate bleeding, while occasionally I would step in to prevent the transection of major structures.

The proper plane is a millimeter over, I thought as one Chief resident struggled through a radical neck dissection.

Don't cut that, as I stayed a junior resident's hand which was in the process of mobilizing the common bile duct, mistaking it for the cystic duct.

And so I retracted and exposed as best I could, helping Dr.J as he slowly separated the stomach from the spleen and other surrounding structures.

The anesthesiologist peered over the drapes. "He's a bit cold; I'm getting a temp of 94.5. How much more do you have to do?"

Quite a bit. Just divide the lesser omentum and get to work on the G-E junction, ran through my head.

At that moment, Dr. Di, the Chief, stuck his head in. "Are you ready for me yet?" he asked.

"We've almost got the stomach mobilized," Dr. J lied.

"What have you been doing for the last 3 ½ hours?" The Chief wondered out loud.

"He's even colder," the anesthesia attending chimed in. "Temp is 94."

"You know," the Chief decided, "we need to stop while we can and warm him up. We'll have to finish tomorrow."

No arguments were forthcoming from me or Dr. J. We closed him up and wheeled him to the Recovery Room. He was kept intubated and sedated as we covered him with blankets which were topped off by a warming blanket. His core temp had fallen to 93.5 by the time he had settled in the Recovery room . I was given the task of sitting with him until he was stable.

He was scheduled for his second stage procedure the following day.

Surgery in two stages or extending beyond 24 hours is not unheard of. The Whipple Procedure, which is a pancreatoduodenectomy, and is performed for tumors in the head of the pancreas, was originally performed as two separate procedures. At the time it was thought to be too extensive to be completed in one sitting. There was a time when surgery for aortoenteric fistulas was staged. In this condition a communication has developed between the bowel, usually the third or fourth part of the duodenum and the aorta. Such a fistula leads to massive GI bleeding, as one might expect. Untreated aorto enteric fistula has a mortality of 100%. The two-step procedure was done to decrease the risk of infection of the new graft which is placed in a, presumably, contaminated field. Unfortunately, mortality was high as the infected aortic closure, under high arterial pressure with the blood pounding against the closed aortic stump, often broke down, which resulted in sudden death for the poor ptient.. Immediate reconstruction is the norm in these modern times. Other complicated reconstructive surgeries may take extended periods of time, such as separation of conjoined twins, which often requires a team approach and surgery over a period of days.

Moose, therefore, was not breaking any new ground.

It was not very difficult to warm him. A combination of warming blankets, fluid warmers, and warmed inspired gases brought his temperature up to a toasty 98.7 in short order. Moose was kept sedated and intubated overnight, with his planned return to surgery the next morning at seven thirty.

Moose was back in the OR by 7:25. The Chief was scrubbed and waiting, determined to avoid the events of the previous day. Moose was positioned on the OR table and, once again, his abdomen was opened. There were no surprises. A moderate amount of the expected serosanguinous fluid was aspirated and the stomach was untwisted, but otherwise all was well.

"Come on in here," Dr. Di said to me. "Help Dr. J."

Under the Chief's watchful eye, the esophagus was dissected away from the esophageal hiatus which brought us into Moose's chest, in the mediastinum, behind the heart and between the lungs.

"There's the tumor," Dr. J announced as the esophagus was lifted off the vertebral column. The hard mass within the esophagus extended above the level of the carina, which is where the trachea divides into the two main bronchi.

Time to open the chest.

"Time to open the chest," Dr. Di announced, echoing my thought.

Dr. Di stepped into my spot, relegating me to second assistant.

They didn't do a classic right posterolateral thoracotomy; rather it was more of an anterolateral approach. The lung was mobilized and retracted away from the esophagus. The pleura over the esophagus and the tumor was opened and esophagus was exposed. There was normal esophagus just below the level of the azygos vein, which meant that at least 2/3 of the esophagus needed to be removed.

"Try to remove some of the mediastinal tissue around the esophagus, in case the tumor has grown through the wall," the Chief instructed.

The surgery moved quickly on this second day, maybe due to the Chief's steadying presence, maybe just because the difficult tedious part was done the day before. The esophagus with its nasty cancer was in the bucket in a little more than an hour. Next the mobilized stomach was brought from the abdomen, through the diaphragm at the esophageal hiatus, and into the mediastinum.

Thus, the stomach replaces the esophagus, elongating from a wine skin shaped storage organ into a passive tube.

"Now, cut a hole in the stomach surface the size of a nickel," the Chief instructed.

Dr. J looked up at me and I smiled. Two days before he had commented that he had studied a dime and a quarter.

"Dr. Di always says to make the gastrotomy either dime-sized or quarter-sized," he's said.

Hope Dr. J knows what a nickel looks like.

He managed to make an appropriate-sized opening in the stomach and the anastomosis proceeded without a hitch. I closed the chest with Dr. J as the Chief scrubbed out. We added a feeding jejunostomy tube, closed the abdomen, and Moose was back in the Recovery Room, still on a ventilator, but otherwise quite well.

As the fourth-year resident it was my job to manage Moose through his postoperative recovery, but under the watchful eyes of the Chief and Dr. J. I was on call that night and checked him every few hours. There was little to check. He was rock stable. He was easily weaned from the ventilator and extubated the following day and out of the ICU on the second day.

I got to know Moose as he spent the next ten days gradually recovering from his two-day surgical affair.

"I was in Vietnam, drafted into the Army," he recounted. "I spent two years battling mud and heat and bugs, fighting for a people who didn't care if they won or lost. I started drinking over there and just kept at it when I got home. I was so angry about everything. My family tried to help but, I was such a son of a bitch they kicked me out. The VA didn't help. I was out on the street, drinking, working the occasional odd job, drinking more. Three years ago I landed in the hospital after passing out in the middle of winter. They said I was really cold that time, too.

"A nurse felt sorry for me I guess and got me into rehab. She was a real angel. Susan was her name. She wasn't much to look at, but she cared about me. I decided it was time to get better, for her sake. She was religious and tried to convert me, but I had too much pride... and anger. But, I went through rehab and got sober. She used to come and visit me a couple of times a week. She said I was her personal project. I didn't want to let her down so I finished the program.

"When I got out I went to see her at the hospital. The unit clerk told me she had taken a medical leave of absence. I went to her apartment and found her. She gave me a big hug, but I could tell she'd been crying.

" 'I've got cancer,' " she said. " 'Stage four they tell me...'

"I didn't hear much else of what she said. All I know is that less than two months later she was gone. Before she died she did tell me something.

" 'Make something of yourself. You're not stupid. Go to school, learn to be or do something. Someday... someday, repay the gift you've been given.'

"I was never quite sure what she meant, but I've tried to repay. Deep down I truly believe that God gave my life back to me, but took Susan in exchange. Now I've reached the point where I can repay and I have cancer. You know I'm supposed to graduate from Seminary next month. Tell me Dr. G, will I get the opportunity to share everything I've learned?"

I stared at his face and then at the ceiling.

"I... don't know," I responded. "Doctors get asked questions like that all the time. How much longer? I never know. Two months? Two years? Ten years? Live your life as if there are no tomorrows? Or ten thousand?"

Moose recovered uneventfully. His pathology revealed no spread to lymph nodes and he was able to swallow without difficulty. He had already gained ten pounds at his follow up clinic appointment.

I saw him one more time about six months later. He was up to 145 pounds and was preparing to leave on a mission trip to Asia. He wouldn't give me any other details. He walked away with a smile on his face.

I think Susan was proud of him.

RAT

It was 4:45 on a Wednesday afternoon, clinic had just finished and I'd be on my way home in fifteen minutes, unless…

"Beeep… Beeep… Beeep"

Rats, it's the emergency room.

"Dr. Gelber, we've got an 85-year-old lady from the county nursing home with a distended abdomen. Could you come and take a look at her?"

So much for going home on time. You think they could have waited fifteen minutes?

I made my way to the surgical side of the ER and found Madge. She was a wrinkled old lady, weighed in at 102 pounds, white hair, black glasses, which magnified sharp blue eyes. Her most distinguishing feature at that moment was a belly that was the size of a medicine ball.

"Hello, Ms. W, I'm Dr. Gelber. How long has your abdomen been so blown up?"

"Glad to know you, Dr. Gelber. Call me Madge. This old belly's been growing for the last five days. I think it's a boy."

"Well, Madge, I think we'll need to deliver it soon," I answered. "Are you having any pain, nausea or vomiting?"

Her look turned a bit serious as she answered, "Mostly pressure, not really pain, and a little nausea. And, I haven't pooped in a week."

"Passing anything out? Gas, diarrhea?"

"Nope, not a toot or tweet for five days."

She had a collection of associated medical problems, typical for your average octogenarian. She had a little hypertension, a bit more congestive heart failure, atrial fibrillation, myocardial infarction a year ago, previous hysterectomy, nothing unusual, but enough to cause the cardiologist to say she was at considerable risk for complications. She had mild abdominal tenderness, but her abdomen was tight as a ripe watermelon and about the same size. Her heart was beating at a rate of 124, blood pressure was 85/50.

Plain abdominal X-Rays revealed massively dilated colon. In particular, the cecum (first part of the colon) measured eighteen centimeters in diameter, well beyond the 12-centimeter diameter when one begins to worry about it bursting.

I called my Chief resident, Dr. J, who deferred to the Chief on call, Dr. B, who came to see the patient and then disappeared. In the meantime I did all the paper work to get Madge admitted and prepared to go to the OR.

Her diagnosis was acute large bowel obstruction.

"At last I get to be around some young blood," she commented as I finished my H&P. "All the men at AHP (the nursing home) are wet noodles, if you get my drift; you know, soft and limp. Maybe, when I'm better, you can show me around the hospital, Dr. G?"

"Of course, but let's get you well first. But, I don't think my wife would appreciate me carrying on."

"She'd never know. Besides, I don't see any wedding ring."

I glanced at my naked finger.

"I don't wear it. Too much taking it off and putting it on. I'd lose it in a week."

Dr. B returned and he said a cecostomy was in order, under local anesthesia.

"I guess you talked to the Chief?" I asked.

Our Chairman, Dr. Di, was a staunch proponent of cecostomy in this situation.

We took her up to surgery and performed the cecostomy, which means decompressing her cecum, the first part of the colon, by placing a tube into it under local anesthesia. The cecum was massively distended with the muscle fibers of the outer layer split apart by the distension, but there was no gangrene or perforation. It was the size of a volley ball. After it was decompressed it looked much healthier. The tube was left connected to a drainage bag and Madge went to the ICU.

Her journey was just beginning.

Over the next forty eight hours she stabilized. Her vital signs, renal function, lab abnormalities all normalized. She was ready to embark on the next stage of her odyssey.

The next step was to figure out the cause of her severe distention. Based on the tests that had been done, the assumption was that she had a mechanical obstruction on the left side of the colon. The most likely causes would be an obstructing tumor or narrowing secondary to diverticulitis. There was an outside possibility she had suffered from Ogilvie's syndrome, otherwise called colonic pseudobstruction, although the initial X-Rays were more suggestive of a mechanical cause.

She was wheeled from the ICU to Radiology where she underwent a barium enema (BE), a test where a radiopaque dye is instilled into the colon and X-Rays are taken at various points. This provides information as to the length, contour of the colon, demonstrating areas of narrowing (stricture) or dilation. Large tumors also can be seen with this test. Madge's BE revealed an abrupt termination of the column of dye in the distal sigmoid colon.

"She's going to need another operation," I told Dr. B.

"Try to prep her using the cecostomy and we'll try to do her surgery in three or four days.

It fell on me and my junior residents and interns to begin to flush her colon with saline every few hours, attempting to clean the abundance of stool trapped within the obstructed colon. The hope was that a clean colon would allow for a single stage resection and anastamosis, avoiding a colostomy and the necessity that she wear a bag.

It was a tedious job. Instill a few hundred cc's of saline and let it drain, add some more and let it drain. At first it seemed hopeless as we kept getting some light brown saline, but little else.

Through it all, Madge managed to keep her sassy edge.

"You know, Dr. G, when I'm all better and back at the home you should come and see. I've got my own room and it's so cold and lonely at times. All the men there are just wrinkled old prunes."

"Let's just get you well first, Madge," I answered.

"Oh, I'm not worried about that. You doctors here are so hard working and caring and conscientious.

Some are pretty sexy, too. I know I'll be back on the dance floor in no time."

"Were you a dancer, Madge?"

"Third prize in the Queens borough ballroom dance off, 1919. Leon and me knocked them over with our cha cha cha. Poor Leon, he was killed a few years later; run over by a horse. He was the love of my life, definitely not a dried up prune or a wet noodle, if you get my drift."

I smiled at her as I finished my flushing of her colon.

"One of my interns will be back a couple of hours. Sorry about Leon."

She didn't answer. She was staring off at nothing, a smile on her face, lost in memories of Leon and happier days.

After four days of flushing and draining, flushing and draining, we pronounced Madge clean. By *we* I meant my Chief resident, the Chairman of Surgery, myself, the second-year resident, the intern, four ICU nurses, the custodian, and two cockroaches who called the ICU home. Her surgery was scheduled for the next morning.

It was a big event. Dr. B was operating with the chairman, with the intern and second-year resident on hand to provide proper retraction. I was left out to hold down the fort in the rest of the hospital, but I managed to hover around the OR to see what was happening.

The surgery started uneventfully, but, as the colon was examined, the surgical team was greeted by a left colon full of solid stool. The plan for a single-stage resection and anastamosis faded away in a column of poop as they went to plan B.

Madge's sigmoid colon was resected, the end was brought out to the skin as a colostomy and the distal colon was closed off and left in the pelvis, a so called Hartmann's pouch.

Madge came through the surgery without a hitch and was wide awake and ready to flirt when I saw her on afternoon rounds.

"Did you guys give me a nice flat tummy? I want to look good in my string bikini this summer," she quipped.

"You're already nothing but skin and bones," I answered, "but you do have a colostomy now, at least for a while."

She gave us a pout and look of disappointment, followed by a shrug of her shoulders as we continued on rounds. She had completed stage two of her journey.

Her recovery was uneventful and she was back tormenting the male residents of the nursing home in a little more than a week. She came back to the clinic a week later where she was seen by one of the interns.

"An ole lady named Madge is asking about you, Dr. G," Intern reported. "She says you missed ballroom night at the nursing home."

I made my way into her room.

"I really can't dance, Madge," I confessed. "Dr. B, now he can dance."

"Well, I guess we can skip the dancing and go straight to bed," she propositioned.

"I think you're more than I can handle, Madge."

And, she went on her way.

She made a second appearance in the clinic a month later, looking quite well, eating, walking, she even gained three pounds.

"When can I get rid of this shit bag?" she asked.

She was now about six weeks post op and she still had the cecostomy tube, which was clamped.

"Let's get your colon checked and then we can think about reversing the colostomy," I explained.

"Good, the sooner the better. Even the old prunes at the home won't give me the time of day with this bag."

I set her up for a colonoscopy the following week, to be done by me, one of the last colonoscopies I ever performed.

As she was wheeling back to the endoscopy suite, she remarked: "You really know how to show a girl a good time."

I smiled, "We'll take good care of you Madge and we'll get you all put back together as soon as we can."

"I like a man who whispers sweet nothings…" and she was out.

The colonoscopy was uneventful, revealing diverticular disease in the descending and proximal sigmoid colon. She was scheduled for reversal of her colostomy ten days hence.

"We'll leave her cecostomy for now. It may add a bit of protection for her after the colostomy reversal," my Chief decided.

At 7:15 a.m., ten days later, Madge was rolled into OR Room 12. Miss C, our cranky, dour, and very experienced circulator, and Mrs. J, our equally skilled scrub tech, made up our crew along with Dr. B, me, and one of our interns. The chairman, officially the attending surgeon on the case, sat nearby in the OR lounge. Dr. B was in the last month of his residency and was functioning independently, and was acting as teaching resident on this case. I was to be the surgeon of record.

And so it started. A midline incision was made and we entered the abdomen, greeted by a few adhesions to the abdominal wall which were quickly and easily dispatched. The small bowel was examined and packed out of the way. The colon leading to the colostomy was identified and freed from scar tissue. All that remained was to find the other end of the colon, dissect enough of it so that the two ends could be connected.

It was like running into a stone wall. Madge's pelvis, where the elusive segment of colon resided, was socked in, a mass of adhesions with tissues more resembling concrete than colon.

Where's the colon?

Where's the bladder?

Where are the ureters?

Where, oh where will I dissect next?

"Let's find the ureters first," I announced to no one in particular.

"Good plan," Dr. B responded.

Starting higher up in the abdomen, away from the dense mass of pelvic scar, I began my search. The proximal colon which led to her colostomy was freed from adhesions first. Behind was a mass of small bowel. I commenced the tedious dissection of this small bowel.

"Do you really need to free up all the small bowel?" Dr. B asked.

"You know the rules: Either you leave it all alone or cut away all the adhesions," I recited.

"Ok, Ok," he answered.

Like the barber/surgeons of old, I began to snip and trim, starting where it was easy and then moving along centimeter by centimeter until, an hour and a half later, all the small bowel was free.

This actually was very helpful. Some of the bowel, as expected, had occupied the pelvis and now it was liberated and safely tucked away in the upper abdomen.

(I have to comment on my terminology, specifically the term *liberated*. It's a bit tongue-in-cheek. I remember reading an operative note for a colon resection. The surgeon dictated that, "The splenic flexure was liberated..." I immediately had visions of colons running through the streets chanting, "I'm free, I'm free..." the term *liberated* in this context always brings a smile to my face.)

Progress was slowly being made. With small bowel out of the way, the ureter was easily identified. The foley balloon was palpable within the bladder and careful dissection behind the bladder revealed a staple line; the staples within the closed off end of the colon.

"I think I just need to dissect enough to be sure that there is only colon, no vagina or bladder," I concluded.

My Chief disagreed.

"You need to be sure it is free enough so there is not tension and adequate blood supply," he answered.

I disagreed, believing that the more the distal colon was dissected, the greater the likelihood that blood supply would be compromised or a nearby structure would be injured. But, I complied with his wishes. He was, after all, more senior, more experienced, and had the power to make my life miserable should he so choose.

With the ureters safely in view and the bladder now out of the way, I worked on the colon and rectum.

First, straight down to the sacral prominence, a safe area where there were no vital structures. Then in front of the colon, separating it from the posterior vagina.

"Is this free enough," I wondered out loud, clearly conveying my view that it was more than enough.

I received the desired nod of acquiescence.

The colostomy was quickly freed from the skin, the actual stoma was resected (removed) to provide a clean end to anastamose to the distal colon. It was immediately apparent that the two ends would not meet. More dissection of the left colon was necessary, which meant liberating the splenic flexure of the colon (there's that image again). Once this task was completed the two ends of colon sat comfortably next to each other, both appeared to be pink and healthy and I was satisfied that their connection would heal uneventfully.

"Use the EEA?" I asked, requested, implored.

"Hand sew. You know what they'll say in conference," Dr. B replied, alluding to the required presentation of the case at one, or several, of our weekly meetings where the cases done that week were presented and discussed.

"And, I'll take the heat," he continued, "not you."

"Ok, I'll sew it. But it won't be easy. We're pretty far down in the pelvis."

I did my best to put the two ends back together. First the back wall of interrupted silk sutures, then the inner layer of continuous Vicryl, an absorbable suture material, and, finally, the outer front layer of silk.

Each suture placement was a chore as I endeavored to be precise; to be sure I caught the full thickness of the bowel wall, while not compromising the lumen diameter. When I finally finished, something just didn't feel right.

"You know," I commented, "something isn't right. I just can't be sure that the two ends have come together properly. Do you think the cecostomy will provide some protection for the anastamosis?"

"You know it won't," Dr. B replied.

"Well, I just don't trust my anastamosis. Maybe we should do a proximal colostomy?" I wondered out loud, a bit facetiously.

Dr. B didn't say a word at first. I suspected he was wondering if he should call Dr. Di, who was the official attending on the case.

"I'll be back in minute," he said and he broke scrub.

"Dr. Di agrees. We should do a transverse colostomy," he announced when he returned.

While he scrubbed his hands again, I mobilized the right transverse colon and we created a transverse loop colostomy, fashioned so that it functioned to completely divert the fecal stream away from my pelvic anastamosis. We closed Madge up and she woke up without a problem, after five hours of surgery.

She sailed through the post-operative recovery. Stage Three was over. She still wasn't finished, however. Now she sported a transverse colostomy and the cecostomy was not completely closed either. She was going to need at least one more surgery.

A month later I was walking past one of the exam rooms in the surgery clinic when I heard a familiar voice.

"There goes my young stud," she cackled.

I made an abrupt U-turn and went into the room where Madge was being checked by one of the interns.

"You know I'd be with you in a minute, Madge," I answered, "but I'm spoken for."

"Another broken heart," she replied, "and I'm stuck with dried up prunes. And, I still have to wear this bag."

"Let's see," I mused as I perused her chart, "it's about six weeks from the last surgery. I think we may be able to do something about that in the next few weeks."

I was Chief resident now, so I went to talk with Dr. Di, who agreed Madge could have her next procedure in two or three weeks.

Her visit to clinic that day gave me the opportunity to give her a complete physical exam. Her midline wound was healing well, the colostomy looked pink and healthy, but the cecostomy site still had not closed completely. There was a five millimeter open wound with some mucus draining.

"It's getting smaller," Madge commented. "Doesn't hurt a bit."

She was scheduled for August the seventh, which was in three weeks. Orders were written and she went on her way, with plans to be admitted to the hospital on the sixth, the day before surgery, when she would have all the necessary preoperative preparation.

The big day came and Madge said she would be happy to be rid of the bag. Of course she took the opportunity to offer herself to me one more time.

"After this surgery you must stop by and see me in my room over at the home, Room 202. Every night it's the same routine: dinner, television, the sounds of arteries hardening and saliva dribbling. Come by and see me. We can go dancing."

And she winked at me as she was rolled into Room 12.

This surgery was a straightforward closure of a loop colostomy. The actual surgery was done by my fourth-year resident, with me acting as teaching assistant.

The incision was made around the stoma and the dissection carried down into the subcutaneous tissue.

"Did you take your slow pill today?" I wondered out loud. My junior resident, Dr. T, was moving like a glacier, one cell layer at a time.

"Open your eyes and see," I suggested. "There is a plane of dissection between the colon and the subcutaneous fat. The mesentery and the subq fat look different and, look, God has left a white line which says 'cut here'."

With a bit of guidance, the fascia, the layer below the fat was finally reached.

"Now, dissect along the fascia so that the colon can be liberated (there's that word again)," I instructed.

My words were greeted by a lost stare out into space.

"Right angle clamp, please," I requested.

I hated to do it, that is, take over the dissection, but, poor Madge was not getting any younger.

I dissected the colon free from the fascia using the clamp, allowing my junior resident to cut in between the jaws of the clamp, which provided some semblance of "doing the case."

The colon finally free, it was delivered up into the wound and continuity restored via a two-layered, hand-sewn, side-to-side anastamosis.

"What next?" I asked as the fourth finished tying the final silk suture.

"Put it back inside, close her up, and then make rounds?" he answered.

"Well, some people would consider that a right answer. If I were actually doing the surgery, I would tack some omentum over the sutures lines. It adds an extra layer of protection, although the way Madge handles surgery, I think you could have used paste to put her back together and it would have healed just fine.

The surgery finally done, after four tedious hours, Madge was tucked away in the Post Anesthesia Care Unit and proceeded through another smooth and uneventful recovery.

She did manage to proposition me on a daily basis until she was discharged once again.

I thought she was done with surgery. Four stages for the treatment of a colon obstruction was a bit unusual. One of the frequent discussions/controversies in general surgery was how to handle acute large bowel obstruction. Should it be a one-stage procedure with resection of the offending segment of colon coupled with some sort of on the OR table bowel cleansing, a-two stage procedure with resection of the diseased segment and creation of a temporary diverting colostomy, followed by a second operation to restore colonic continuity, or a three-stage procedure with an initial diverting colostomy, a second operation to remove the cause of the obstruction and then a third procedure to reverse the colostomy.

Dear Madge had undergone four stages.

I saw Madge in the clinic a week later, healing quite well, eating normally, having normal bowel movements, and overall quite satisfied. Her only complaint was persistent drainage from the cecostomy site.

"It should close, just give it some time," I reassured her.

"I'm sure it will, Dr. G," she replied and then she smiled at me. "Of course, It might be best if you came to check on it over at the home a couple of times a month."

I smiled back. Good old, dependable Madge.

"I think your coming to the clinic will be adequate," I answered.

"Stuck with all the old prunes," she murmured.

I saw her again a month later. She was still draining from the cecostomy site. As a matter of fact, the open area looked larger, with a bit of intestinal mucosa poking out.

"It looks like you'll need another surgery to close up the cecostomy," I informed her.

She shrugged her shoulders and nodded her approval. Then, as if sensing some disappointment on my part, she added, "Can I have a private room this visit? One never knows when a handsome young red headed doctor will come calling and try to take advantage of a girl."

I smiled and said, "See you next week."

The surgery came and went off without a hitch. My second-year resident performed the surgery while I acted as teaching assistant.

We dissected around the cecum, following it down to the fascia, cutting away all the scar tissue and, finally, delivering the cecum into the wound. There was a 1.5 cm hole which was closed in two layers, then reinforced with a bit of fat before it was dunked back into its rightful home within the peritoneal cavity. We closed her up and she went to the PACU for the final time, I hoped.

Sure enough, except for shifting her affections from me to the younger and handsomer junior resident, her post-operative recovery was smooth sailing.

"I'm a little disappointed, Madge," I explained to her on the day she was discharged. "You seem to have shifted your amorous affections from me to Dr. K."

"Well, Dr. G, I'm not getting any younger. You had your chance and you blew it. Besides, Dr. K is really hot," she answered.

"Good luck, Madge," I responded. "And, I say this with all affection, but I hope I don't ever see you on my OR table again."

She smiled and nodded her understanding, but then added, "Do you have Dr. K's phone number?"

"You'll have to ask him yourself. I'm sure he'll be around to see you before you leave."

She sighed and then added, "I guess it's back to wet noodles and prunes."

I did see her back in the clinic about a week later, one last time. She healed without a problem and thanked me for helping to save her life.

Her case had been different than most. There was no discussion about one-stage, two-stage, or three-stage procedures.

Madge had undergone a five-stage procedure.

A few weeks later I had a meeting with our chairman, Dr. Di, and I brought up her case.

"Remember Madge, the old lady who had the large bowel obstruction and had the five-stage colon resection?" I asked the chairman.

"She was a rat," he answered, his response taking me by surprise.

"I thought she was very nice," I answered.

"I don't mean a rat, as in James Cagney, 'you dirty rat,' sense," he said in his grandfatherly tone. "No, I meant she's a rat because she could be operated on over and over and never turn a hair."

He explained further.

"Years ago there was an experiment done. A number of rats had surgery, all the same sham operation. After the first operation, some of the rats died. The survivors were operated on a second time and a few more died. The third time a few more. But, after a number of operations some of those rats just went on like nothing happened. You could operate on those rats every week and they wouldn't turn a hair. They just woke up and went on their way.

"Madge was a one of those rats."

A SWEET MAN

He was a sweet man. That's what the Chief said about Adrian. Adrian did have his issues, that's for sure. Number one was that he was yellow. I don't mean yellow in the sense that he was cowardly; quite the opposite was true. Adrian was literally yellow.

That was why he was in our clinic. His skin and eyes were yellow and he had been having abdominal pain. He couldn't eat and had lost almost twenty pounds. Obstructive jaundice was the diagnosis. I put him in the hospital to find out why.

Besides his yellowness, Adrian had other problems. He had been born with cerebral palsy and had spent most of his life in a variety of institutions. Maybe he was a bit slow to collect his thoughts, perhaps his words weren't always clear and his eyes looked a little "off." But, he had a smile that lit up the room. And when he smiled his eyes had a little twinkle that said, "I know I look a little different, but looks are nothing. It's what's in the heart that counts."

He and the Chief hit it off almost immediately, even though they were worlds apart intellectually, socially, and in every other way. The Chief saw something special in Adrian; call it purity or sincerity.

I, on the other hand, had to tend to business; in this case, the task was finding out why poor Adrian was yellow and what could be done to fix him.

The history offered some clues. Adrian had suffered repeated episodes of upper abdominal pain and back pain with nausea. The pain lasted a few hours, occurred at all hours of the day, but was worse at night.

So far, classic gallbladder disease with episodes of biliary colic.

Physical exam revealed scleral icterus and not much else. Specifically, there was no abdominal mass and neither the liver nor spleen was enlarged.

Lab tests were significant for a total bilirubin of 9.3, Alkaline phosphatase was 815. CBC, electrolytes, BUN, Creatinine, and everything else was essentially normal. Ultrasound revealed gallstones and a dilated common bile duct.

Adrian was a classic case of chronic cholecystitis, cholelithiasis, and choledocholithiasis, which means he had pain secondary to stones in the gallbladder and common bile duct. Surgery would be the proper treatment.

The time was 1989. Laparoscopic Surgery had not yet hit the United States in any big way. There was no MRCP and ERCP's were not done if the patient was going to need surgery anyway. Besides, I was a resident, this was a teaching hospital, and Cholecystectomy and Common Bile Duct Exploration was a good case; it was what we called a "Complex Interchangeable Case." A minimum of sixty such cases were needed to sit for the boards. And, to top it off, this particular surgery, specifically Common Bile Duct Exploration, was one of the Chief's favorite types of operation.

I scheduled Adrian during my regular operating time, which was on Thursday, three days hence. I notified the Chief and thought everything was set.

That's when the problems started. Not with Adrian, he was fine waiting a couple of days. He greeted us every morning with his special smile. He told us how much he liked the food and how comfortable the bed was. He waved goodbye as we left and told us how he looked forward to seeing us on afternoon rounds.

No, it wasn't Adrian. It was me and a sudden flurry of very sick and complicated patients. Gregory had a mass in the right middle lobe of his lung and needed a resection. Thomas had a mass in the left upper lobe of his lung and *he* needed a resection. Jesse had stomach cancer; Johnny had colon cancer; Phil had a chest wall mass. All were in the hospital and all needed complex surgery. So much work, so little time. And the Chief was involved with not only Adrian, but Gregory and Thomas.

I must point out that at the county hospital each Chief resident is allotted a certain amount of OR time. I had Room 12 on Tuesday, Thursday, and Friday. Scheduled cases had to be finished by 3:00 p.m. I would need to do some wheeling and dealing to find the time to do this windfall of Complex Interchangeable Cases.

I called my co-chief resident on the Trauma service and borrowed his time on Wednesday, and I rescheduled a few other smaller cases. Because of scheduling conflicts with other attending surgeons, Adrian's surgery was moved to Friday. Finally, I went up to the office to tell the Chief about the change in schedule.

He was not happy.

"I cancelled an important meeting to do that surgery. Do not *ever* take me for granted. Change it back," he almost shouted, the first and last time he ever raised his voice at me.

A bit sheepishly, I got on the phone with scheduling some of the other attending surgeons and the other Chief residents, and managed to put things back so that Adrian's case with the Chief was back on Thursday. Of course, the other Chief residents, feigning helpfulness, said that they would be willing to make the sacrifice and do one or more of these complicated surgeries for me.

Just to be helpful.

Such help I did not need.

It took a bit of finagling, begging, and dealing, but I managed to get all my cases scheduled in a timely manner, fulfill all my necessary duties, and keep the Chief happy.

Adrian waited patiently. He remained yellow, but otherwise was well. On rounds the following day he was doing his best to help out some other patients as well as the hospital staff. We found him emptying the wastebasket in his room into the janitor's larger trash can. He called the nurses when his roommate's IV ran out. He bought food from the vending machines on the floor and shared his Frito's and Cheetoh's with the other patients.

The day before surgery I sat down at his bedside and explained his surgery to him. I presented the alternatives, risks, benefits, and all the other details as simply and clearly as I could. He listened intently, nodding his head once in a while, but I was never sure if he truly understood. When I finished I asked him if he had any questions.

"You know," he began, "it would be really nice if I could get a job here after my surgery. Maybe, I could sweep up or take out the trash."

And he smiled his sweet smile.

"Let's get you better first," I answered. "I don't have much influence over such things, but the Chief might be able to help. I'll talk to him."

"Thank you, thank you," he responded and his smile grew even larger.

There are parts of being a doctor which have nothing to do with physical wellbeing. For example, I have a patient who had rectal cancer many years ago. I remember before his surgery that his biggest concern was getting back to work, which was janitorial. He was the sole support for his family. Neither he nor his wife spoke English, yet they managed. He told me that the worst thing was to be unproductive. He needed to be doing something which helped others, even if it was just mopping floors.

"Clean floors," he told me through an interpreter, "are important to a hospital. My floors are the cleanest."

And, I believed they were.

Adrian, I'm sure, had similar beliefs. He wanted to be productive. He wanted to look at a floor or an empty waste basket and feel pride in a job well done. Yes, he suffered from a chronic infirmity, but this so called disability was in no way an impediment to his productivity.

The question was: "When should I bring it up to the Chief?"

Dr. Di, the Chief, was already annoyed with me. Should I do it now, figuring two annoyances at the same time will pass sooner than one after another? Or, maybe, wait until he calms down and forgets about my recent transgression. He likes Adrian; I'm sure he would be happy to help out one of his patients.

After considerable mental deliberation I decided to bring the issue up while we were operating. During the surgery Adrian would be center stage and doing all things possible to help *him* would be foremost in all our minds.

Finally, Adrian's big day came.

The Chief waited in our tiny lounge while I began the surgery with one of the junior residents. The Chief always preferred midline incisions, even for gallbladder surgery. He poked his head into the room shortly after we started and scrubbed in as the gallbladder was passed to the scrub tech.

Adrian was very thin with a paucity of intraabdominal fat. The Structures of the Porta Hepatis: bile duct, hepatic artery and portal vein stood out. The bile duct was very dilated, almost two centimeters in diameter. This was about three times the normal size of six to eight millimeters.

"Looks pretty obvious, don't you think Chief?" I asked, pointing to the bile duct.

"You still need to follow the rules," he responded.

"I know, I was just testing you," I shot back; I'm sure he smiled at me from behind his mask.

The rule was that the bile duct always should be aspirated with a needle before it is opened. It was considered bad form to make an incision in a structure, assuming it was the common bile duct, only to discover it was the portal vein. Bad form for the surgeon and especially bad for the patient.

With 23-gauge needle and syringe in hand, I aspirated the structure which I was sure was the CBD and was happy to see the syringe fill up with yellow fluid. I put stay sutures in the duct and made my incision. Bile and a big stone popped out.

Maybe this won't be too difficult. Be careful. Don't say anything or you'll jinx yourself.

"Choledochoscope," the Chief requested. As we were waiting for Jeanette, the scrub tech, to set up the scope, the Chief looked up at me and then down at Adrian's abdominal viscera.

"You know," he began in his slightly gruff, grandfatherly way, "when you die and go to that big operating room in the sky, all your cases will be like this."

This was the second time during my residency that the Chief made this observation; the other was on a similar case in a very thin, young, and healthy woman. And, I knew exactly what he meant.

Surgery like Adrian's were the Chief's favorite type of case. But, this particular surgery was shaping up to be interesting, but without the struggles that we sometimes faced when confronted with a patient who is very obese or has extensive inflammation or scar tissue. All of which can make for very tedious operations. Adrian, in a different way, also proved to be a challenge.

The choledochoscope was finally ready. The Chief preferred the rigid scope. He thought the visualization was better and instrumentation was easier. This scope consisted of an optics portion which was inserted into the bile duct and an eyepiece which was at a right angle to the optical portion. Using this particular choledochoscope required a Kocher maneuver, which meant mobilizing the duodenum, so that downward traction could be exerted to straighten out the duct and allow for inspection of the entire duct.

The Chief inserted this scope through the opening in the bile duct and then handed the scope to me. A stone was clearly visible.

We went to work and fished it out using a stone forceps. The scope went back in and another stone was seen and removed, then another and another. Before long we had ten stones.

"There are more in there," I commented.

"Keep at it," the Chief replied.

Five more stones were removed and there was at least one more.

"This last stone is stuck," I noted. Looking with the scope, we both saw the stone wedged in the duct and I could feel it behind the duodenum.

"I'll try a Fogarty," I decided and the Chief nodded his head in concurrence.

The Fogarty, a catheter with an inflatable balloon on its tip, would not pass beyond the stone. We tried stone forceps, irrigation, another go around with the Fogarty, but that stone did an excellent imitation of a mule and refused to budge.

"If this is what I have to look forward to in Heaven, I hate to think about the alternative," I quipped.

The Chief gave me a look of frustration, then asked, "What's your plan now?"

"The duct is big; I think a choledochoduodenostomy would be best. Adrian has a lot of stones. I wonder if some or all of them formed in the duct, rather than passing from the gallbladder," I explained, offering my reasoning.

"You wouldn't consider a transduodenal sphincteroplasty?" He asked, playing Devil's advocate I suspected.

"With the big duct and so many stones, I think the bypass operation is better," I replied. "Besides, we won't have to worry about a cholangiogram."

These two procedures are similar. But have different potential for complications, short term and long term. A choledochoduodenostomy means anastomosing the duodenum and the common bile duct, thus bypassing the obstructed portion of the duct behind the duodenum. This allows for much improved drainage from the bile duct. A transduodenal sphincteroplasty means approaching the bile duct through the duodenum at the ampulla of Vater. The duodenum is opened and the ampulla, which is where the bile duct and pancreatic duct enter the bowel, is identified. This ampulla is then incised, which opens the sphincter, which is then sutured to the duodenal mucosa. This enlarges the opening between the common bile duct and duodenum.

The latter procedure, in my opinion, is best for impacted stones at the ampulla and short ampullary strictures. The sphincteroplasty is also useful when the bile duct is small, as the biliary bypass procedure is more likely to fail if the duct is less than one centimeter. Long term, the sphincteroplasty is more physiologic and less likely to have the complication of ascending cholangitis, which means infection of the biliary system, which is more common after choledochoduodenostomy.

In Adrian's case, his duct was large and there was concern that the stones may have developed within the common bile duct. Both these facts led me to recommend the choledochoduodenostomy.

The Chief agreed.

I already had a hole in the bile duct. I made an opening in the duodenum and hooked the two together with a minimum of fuss.

While suturing away, I asked the Chief about Adrian.

"Chief," I started, "Adrian asked if he could have a job with the County. Maybe a janitor or something like that. He really will do whatever he can. I think he would be a good worker."

"Such a nice, sweet man," he answered. "You know, it would be the right thing to help him. I'll talk to some of the administrative types."

And that was that.

I finished Adrian's operation in short order and he made a rapid, uneventful recovery, going from yellow to pink over a couple of weeks, when I saw him back in the clinic.

"I haven't forgotten about what you asked," I reminded him as I felt his abdomen. "The Chief spoke with the Hospital CEO and you have an appointment with Human Resources on Friday. Can you make it?"

He gave me his big smile and his eyes shone.

"I'll be there," he answered and he smiled again.

"Wait, before you go, the Chief wants to say hello," I added.

The Chief came from the back and shook Adrian's hand.

"Good luck, Adrian," was all the Chief said and he walked away.

However, I did hear him murmur, "Such a sweet man."

PIZZA BY THE SLICE

I inherited Rollie. Actually, he was more of a gift. I had been with my new group in Houston for about a week and had just been granted temporary privileges.

"Do you think you could take care of a patient for me?" one of my new associates asked.

"Sure," I answered.

I was young, energetic, and eager to impress and be of help to my new, more seasoned partners.

"His name is Rollie. He's got acute pancreatitis, in ICU bed 16," my partner informed me.

"OK."

Right up my alley.

I was fresh from the County hospital in New York. Cases of severe pancreatitis had become a specialty of mine. In the year before moving to Texas I had cared for half a dozen patients with severe, life threatening acute pancreatitis. The Chief had commented that he didn't think any of them would survive, but I guess he was wrong, because each of these severely ill patients completely recovered and walked out of the hospital.

I went to see Rollie, all 365 pounds of him.

"How do you feel?" I asked him.

"Lousy," was his response.

I probably didn't need to ask. Rollie was sprawled out on the hospital bed, diaphoretic, IV's in each arm, an NG tube and Foley catheter in place. His hair was a greasy tousle, his face was flushed and he was huffing and puffing at a rate of 28. The monitors reported a heart rate of 120 and oxygen saturation of 92%. Blood pressure was elevated at 160/90.

He looks sick. Thank you, Dr. H.

"When did you start to feel 'lousy'?" I asked.

"After I ate all that pizza," he reported.

"When was that?"

"Five days ago. I ate 36 slices of pizza and then I got sick with pain in my stomach and back, nausea and vomiting. I've been here since last night and I only feel worse."

"It looks like we're doing everything we can," I answered looking at the IV fluids which were running, at the urine Rollie was producing, and then tapping on his abdomen.

He winced in pain.

"I'll be back in a little while. I'm going to look at the tests they've done so far." I put my hand on his left arm and went to look at his chart.

Abdominal pain for five days, nausea and vomiting, Lipase 1200, Amylase 550, WBC 28,000, H/H 16.5/52, HCO3 17, Glucose 250, etc. etc.

CT scan demonstrated the expected diffuse edema of the pancreas with surrounding inflammation and fluid in the lesser sac extending to around the left kidney.

"All in all, a picture of bad pancreatitis," I remarked out loud.

I went over Rollie's current orders…"NPO, IV at 200cc/hr, pain med, antibiotics, Foley, NG tube…"

Looks appropriate. Now just sit back and wait.

Pancreatitis, particularly early in the course of the disease, is largely wait and see. All a doctor can do is institute optimal supportive care with IV fluids, respiratory support, and medications to control symptoms and treat complications while waiting to see if the disease will progress or resolve. My experience told me that Rollie, if he survived, was in for a long, complicated, and perilous ride.

At least he'll lose some weight. Probably never eat pizza again.

Rollie stayed about the same over the next 72 hours. He continued to require large volumes of IV fluids to maintain adequate vital signs and kidney function. He developed almost every "bad sign" of pancreatitis one could imagine. By the third day he was huffing and puffing at 40 times a minute, but could not maintain his oxygen level and was intubated.

Now, it was a battle for his life.

Based on Ranson's criteria for predicted severity of acute pancreatitis, Rollie's hope for survival was near zero. Fortunately, he had never read these textbooks. Although very ill, he began to stabilize. He was able to maintain his kidney function and I suspect this is what kept him alive.

After six days in the hospital, he went for a repeat CT of the abdomen.

"Multiple pseudocysts, the largest measured 20 cm in diameter, severe peripancreatic inflammation, multiple thickened loops of small and large bowel, no free air, no abscess."

Nothing which surgery will help.

Although my experience was not a prospective randomized double-blind study, I believed that avoiding surgery, or at least waiting until 2-3 weeks into the course of the disease, afforded the best outcomes. Most often surgery became necessary if the patient developed an abscess or necrosis of the pancreas or complications involving surrounding organs such as perforation of the bowel or severe bleeding. So far, none of these had occurred.

Sit tight.

"Don't you think we should drain those pseudocysts?" Dr. Internist asked.

"Only make things worse," I answered.

Dr. Infectious disease consulted Interventional Radiology to aspirate some of the fluid.

I cancelled his order.

"They usually go transgastric," I explained to him, "and all they will do is contaminate the area and turn the pseudocyt into an abscess."

He nodded his head, but I'm not sure he was in agreement.

"Trust me, it's best to continue with the current therapy."

He nodded his head again.

Rollie continued along a sort of smoldering clinical course, not improving much, but also not deteriorating.

He required 60% oxygen to maintain saturation around 95%. His IV fluid needs now were at maintenance levels and his liver and kidney function was normal.

I think he'll make it.

And he improved. Gradually, oh so slowly, his lungs improved. His oxygen requirements fell to 55%, then 50%, 45% and settled at 40%. His GI tract began to function and he was changed from Total Parenteral Nutrition (TPN) to Enteral Feedings via a nasojejunal tube. TPN, which is a means of providing complete nutritional requirements through a central venous catheter, is not truly physiologic, carrying with it the potential for severe infectious and metabolic complications. Enteral feedings, on the other hand, provide nutrition via the GI tract, avoiding most of the potential complications while feeding the sick patient in the way God intended.

Another CT scan revealed that Rollie's "pseudocysts" were evolving. The fluid collections were more defined, the inflammation around the pancreas was much less, the pancreas itself now looked healthy.

No question he has turned the corner. Just keep him away from pizza.

Two weeks later Rollie was eating, walking around, and ready to leave. His weight was now 270 pounds.

He was to follow up with the GI specialist and his newly assigned primary care physician. I hadn't done any surgery, so there was no reason for him to see me.

I had almost forgotten about him when I passed him at the hospital. He didn't look good.

"Rollie, how are you?" I asked stopping him in the hall.

"OK, I guess, I feel sort of weak."

"Not eating any pizza, I hope."

"No, not eating much of anything."

Rollie looked ill, very ill. Pale, sunken eyes, listless manner, all the hallmarks of someone who was wasting away. He almost looked like he was in the final stages of terminal cancer, quite a trick for someone who had been over 350 pounds only a couple of months before.

"Come to my office this afternoon at two. Don't forget. Here's my card. If you don't come, I'll call you."

"OK, Dr. G."

Rollie showed up precisely at two. He now weighed 175 pounds. He was very pale, his heart rate was 110 and his blood pressure was 85/60.

"You need to be in the hospital," I explained. "Something is not right."

Rollie had seen his doctors only one time since his major illness. He was at the hospital that day to visit a friend who had been in a car accident.

"It hurts when I eat," he reported. "I get sick and throw up. All I can do is drink water."

"You look very pale," I told him. "Noticed any blood when you go to the bathroom or had any vomiting of blood?"

"Not that I've noticed. Just pain and nausea."

Rollie had an H/H of 4.5 and 14, severe anemia. Otherwise his lab test looked OK. He was transfused three units of packed red blood cells while he awaited the requisite CT scan. I also called Dr. R, his GI specialist.

"You remember Rollie, big, young kid with bad pancreatitis. The one who ate all that pizza. Well, he's back in the hospital, lost a lot of weight, severely anemic. He may need at least an EGD, maybe a colonoscopy. CT will be done today.

"You'll see him this evening. Good, Thanks."

Dr. R called later, just after I saw the results of Rollie's CT of the abdomen.

"Rollie's been bleeding from gastric varices," we each said, almost in unison.

"I did an EGD this evening and he's got huge gastric varices," Dr. R reported.

"His CT reveals splenic vein thrombosis," I answered. "So gastric varices make sense. His pseudocysts are much smaller."

He's going to need surgery.

Rollie's anemia almost certainly was due to bleeding from these gastric varices. Varices are extremely dilated veins. They are often very thin walled and bleed easily with minimal irritation. What happened in this case is that Rollie's severe pancreatitis caused the splenic vein, which carries blood from the spleen and pancreas to the portal vein, then through the liver and then to the heart, to thrombose, which means it is obstructed. The blood from the spleen and pancreas needs to find new avenues to flow. The pancreas has collateral arterial flow through the vessels called the pancreatoduodenals, but blood from the spleen must take a different route. This almost is always via the short gastric vessels. Normally, blood flows through these short gastric veins into the splenic vein. However, with the splenic vein occluded the flow of blood is reversed and the high flow from the spleen now must pass through the usually small short gastric veins. With time these veins dilated to accommodate the increased flow, but, as a consequence, became fragile and bled very easily.

"I need to take out your spleen," I informed Rollie and I explained the whole scenario.

"We'll do the surgery tomorrow morning, that is, if you want. But, I don't see a lot of alternatives."

"I trust you, Dr. G. I'll see you tomorrow."

At least he's not 365 pounds any more.

Rollie was wheeled into OR four at 10:00 a.m.

What type of incision? Midline? Left subcostal?

I looked over his CT scan again. My concern was not the spleen, rather it was the pseudocysts. Should I do something with them? Or just take care of the problem at hand?

The largest remaining pseudocyst was about 8 cm in diameter and was between the stomach and the pancreas.

Maybe that pseudocyst is why he has pain when he eats.

All the others were small, two centimeters or less.

Left subcostal it is. This was an incision on the left side of the abdomen below and parallel to the lowest rib. Such an incision would allow excellent access to the spleen, stomach and the distal part of the pancreas and would allow me to drain the largest pseudocyst if necessary.

Once Rollie was prepped and draped, I made my incision.

Get the colon out of the way first.

Most of the time when I operate on the pancreas, spleen, or stomach, my first order of business is to get the transverse colon out of my way. In Rollie's case it was the splenic flexure of the colon, which is the most distal part of the transverse colon, which can be bothersome.

Just get the colon out of the way so you don't have to worry about injuring it. Careful, there's a lot of fibrosis, stay close to the spleen.

In this case, where there was considerable scarring from the recent pancreatitis, it was more prudent to dissect the spleen free from the colon, rather than vice versa. This may sound like a game of semantics, but there is a difference which is that dissecting the spleen means little or no manipulation of the colon, while the spleen is retracted and its attachments to the colon divided.

Next I approached the pancreas which was easily palpable, hard and fibrotic, not its usual soft and spongy consistency. I continued my dissection close to the spleen, leaving the pancreas alone, careful not to injure it. This brought me to the hilum of the spleen, where the splenic artery and vein entered the organ.

I don't need to worry about the vein, but the artery may be a challenge.

Indeed, the tissue at the hilum was a hard mass of fibrotic and inflamed scar.

Maybe the CT will help.

I studied the CT again. The splenic artery could be seen in the posterior aspect of the pseudocyst.

So, if I enter the pseudocyst right behind the stomach it should be safe.

Slowly, carefully, I incised over the pseudocyst and after dividing about a centimeter of thick scar, I was rewarded with an oozing of thick greenish fluid. I cleaned all this out and was able to trace the course of the fibrotic pancreas and feel for the location of the splenic artery.

Back to the spleen.

It was much easier to continue my dissection now that the pseudocyst was drained. From here it was just clamp, clamp, cut, clamp, clamp, cut, and in five minutes the spleen was in the bucket.

What should I do with the remnant of the pseudocyst?

That was a good question. The optimal treatment for a pancreatic pseudocyst which requires surgery is internal drainage, which means connecting the cyst to the stomach or small bowel. Such a procedure requires the cyst have an adequate capsule so that the sutures used to make the connection have something to hold. If the capsule is thin or if there is no capsule then external drainage with a large drainage tube is more appropriate.

External drainage for Rollie.

After all the dissection which was necessary to remove the spleen, there wasn't much of the pseudocyst left, certainly not enough to hook up to any of the surrounding bowel. I left a big closed suction drain in front of the pancreas, just in case any fluid wanted to reaccumulate in that area.

Rollie made a remarkable recovery. He felt much better, was able to eat and was ready to leave five days after surgery.

I went to discharge him around lunch time.

He was eating pepperoni pizza.

A HORSE IS A HORSE OF COURSE

Jeremy was a cowboy in the rodeo. He also was responsible for keeping me up for most of three nights in a row. He was the fortunate survivor of a run-in with a very angry horse.

Animals are supposed to be our friends, at least dogs and cats, horses, pigs, and cows. Some birds, the occasional snake, and even tarantulas have been companions to humanity. Our encounters with these domesticated beasts are supposed to bring pleasure, happiness, and feelings of wellbeing.

Except, when they don't.

One patient of mine, Melvin, was set upon unmercifully by two feral dogs, losing large chunks of skin and muscle from each leg and one arm before the beasts could be restrained. Sandy was a young lady tattooed from head to toe. She had a pet python who mistook her for his dinner one day and tried to swallow her whole. I see half a dozen patients every year with fever and painful swollen lymph nodes secondary to cat scratch disease. Bird bites, tarantula bites, dog bites, and so many other bites have made it into the hospital over the years.

But Jeremy; he stands out. Maybe it's because he showed up in the ER very early in my career in private practice; maybe it was the running battle between his divorced parents, maybe it was the conversation with

Dr. Red Duke, or the lack of sleep I accumulated over the four days it took to stabilize him. Probably all of the above combined to make him one of my more memorable disasters.

I had been out in private practice for about four months and I still had the feeling of invincibility common to surgeons as they leave the safety of residency and head out to save the real world. It was 11:00 p.m. when the phone rang.

"Dr. G, this is Dr. F in the ER. I've got an 18-year-old man here who got kicked in the right side by a horse. His heart rate is 130 and BP is 90. There's a big area of swelling on his right side. He's on his way to CT as we speak."

"OK, thanks, I'll be in to see him," I answered. I turned to my wife.

"I need to go to work," I said.

"Surgery?" she asked.

"Don't know. I hope it's nothing major."

I pulled on some clean scrubs and left.

Jeremy was just finishing his CT as I arrived. As he was wheeled back to the ER, I scrolled through his scan.

Broken rib, looks like a pretty big subcapsular hematoma of the liver, not much else.

This was my reading of the scan, but usually I was pretty accurate, as I had spent the last two years of my residency reading abdominal CT's with the senior Radiology residents.

The Radiologist's official reading was in agreement.

Jeremy was awake and alert, complaining of pain in his right side. He had been competing in a local rodeo and one of the horses decided nobody was going to ride him and decided to vent his anger on Jeremy, delivering a solid kick squarely to Jeremy's right side where there was a big bruise. I was sure I could make out the imprint of a horseshoe. Certainly not lucky for Jeremy.

Jeremy's Dad was at his bedside showing nothing but the proper concern. Mom and fireworks would show up later.

Jeremy stabilized after a couple of liters of IV fluids and I decided surgery was not needed at this time. I tucked him away in the ICU and was back in bed by 2:00 a.m.

Later in the morning, Jeremy was looking fairly stable. Heart rate was around 110, blood pressure was 110/70, urine output and oxygen saturation were good. His hgb had dropped for 14 to 10.5.

"Looks like he's pretty stable," I reassured his dad.

"His mother will be happy," he replied.

"I haven't met his mother yet," I answered.

"She's been away on a business trip. She's flying in this afternoon and will be here later."

"Oh, well I guess I'll meet her later. I'll check on him this evening," I added and I left to attend to other sick people.

A few hours later a message came to call the ICU regarding lab results.

"Jeremy's hemoglobin has dropped to seven," the nurse reported, "and his heart rate is 125. Blood pressure is 100/60."

"Give him two units of Packed RBC's," I ordered.

Looks like he's going to need surgery. I hate operating on the liver.

That was the truth. I loved operating on the biliary system, pancreas, and everything else around the liver, but the liver itself was one of my least favorite organs to work on.

Maybe it's because you can't really take it out. Every other intra-abdominal organ could be removed if necessary, its functions then assumed by other organs or replaced with medication. The esophagus can be replaced by a segment of colon or even small bowel, stomach can be reconstructed, much of the bowel can be resected with impunity, dialysis can replace kidneys if necessary, there are insulin and enzymes for the pancreas, but the liver is different.

No other organ does its job, metabolizing bile salts, detoxifying noxious chemicals, releasing stored glucose along with so many other functions. Transplantation is the only truly viable treatment alternative if a liver fails or has to be removed. I was not really anticipating having to remove all of Jeremy's liver. My point is that the bleeding needed to be stopped and sometimes this can be problematic when dealing with the liver.

I considered repeating his CT scan, but decided that this wouldn't change the inevitable.

So the blood transfusion was started and he was scheduled for surgery. It was 6:30 when I went to explain the situation to his parents, both Mom and Dad now present.

"You let him ride in the rodeo. I told you to stop it," I heard Mom hissing loudly.

"He's an adult. I can't live his life," Dad replied in more of a whisper.

"You could if you were more of a man," Mom answered, the hissing growing louder.

I took that moment to interrupt and introduce myself to Mom.

"I'm Dr. G, I'm pleased to meet you," I began, addressing Mom. "I think you know that Jeremy needs surgery. I'd hoped he would stabilize, but that hasn't happened."

"I'd like to send him to the Med Center," she stated.

"That would be fine with me," I answered, "but he's not stable at the moment. He really needs to go to surgery. I think we're just about ready to start. Afterwards, when he is stable, we can try to arrange for a transfer."

She looked at me with an expression which said, "You better take care of my Jeremy or else…"

I left the worried family and met the OR crew as they began to wheel Jeremy down the hall from ICU to the OR.

"Don't worry," I reassured him, "we're going to take good care of you." This has been my standard line to worried patients over the years, short and to the point, but very effective.

Jeremy was fairly stable as I made my long midline incision. His heart rate was 120, BP 110/60.

Upon entering the abdomen I was greeted by blood, blood, and more blood, dark blood wafting up from between loops of slightly pale bowel. There was more blood around the liver, redder, fresher, along with large congealed clots.

We, that is myself and my assistant, scooped out all the blood and began by packing "laps" all around the abdomen, starting with right upper quadrant around the liver, then around the spleen and in the lower abdomen.

The money is on the liver. At least I don't see a lot of active bleeding.

I pulled the packs from the lower abdomen. This area was pristine, no active bleeding, no hematoma. Next I "ran the bowel" which means I checked the small bowel from its beginning at the Ligament of Treitz until it terminated in the cecum. No injury. The packs were pulled from around the spleen. The left upper quadrant was also spotless; without bleeding or injury.

Time to work.

I gingerly removed the packs from around the liver. There was adherent clot over most of the right lobe with a laceration into the parenchyma and a small amount of oozing of red blood. The capsule of the liver had been disrupted over most of the right lobe.

Maybe just leave a drain? No, he's been bleeding. I definitely need to do something.

I left the clotted blood which coated the denuded liver surface in place and approached the laceration. This was a crevice which ran from the mid superior right lobe to the lateral and inferior aspect of the liver. Bright red blood was slowly welling up and then running down the liver's surface. Carefully, carefully, I put my hand behind the liver and gingerly lifted the right lobe; this brought the laceration closer to me so that I could actually see what I was doing. I packed laps behind the liver which helped hold it in place. I divided the right triangular ligament, which is a peritoneal attachment holding the right lobe. This allowed me to bring the laceration even closer. Now I could see into the depths of the liver, clean out the clot under direct vision, find what was bleeding, and stop it.

I hope.

I began by washing away the clot, irrigating it with saline, doing my best to cause as little disturbance as possible so as not to stir up new bleeding.

What's happening?

My thoughts preceded my words.

"Is there a problem?" I asked the anesthesiologist. "All of a sudden everything is bleeding."

Indeed, the surface of the liver was now a continuous ooze of blood which was filling up the belly. The laceration was briskly filling up with bright red blood. The trickle had become a flood.

"Nothing's changed...wait, how did that happen?" the anesthesiologist replied.

"How did what happen?" I inquired, a sense of urgency in my voice.

"His temp is 93.5. I've only given him 2 units of blood, but something has caused his temp to drop. I don't know how long it will take to warm him."

How did he get so cold? Maybe a transfusion reaction? Just pack him for now, get him warmed up, and then come back and fix the problem.

The commotion at the head of the table faded away as I tuned out everything and concentrated on the problem at hand.

"Laps, a bunch of them," I ordered, the level of my voice rising only slightly.

I packed laps into and around the lacerated liver, holding pressure, and then packing more until they stayed dry.

I closed his belly quickly and we rolled him back to the ICU. His blood pressure was 100/60, heart rate 110, temp 92.7.

I rushed through the immediate post op tasks of dictation and orders and then went to face his worried family.

I found Mom and Dad in heated discussion.

"Would you believe it?" Mom stated as she turned to me. "Wonder man here has an insurance plan that doesn't cover 'animal-related injuries.' What kind of insurance is that?"

"One of the questions was about animal-related activities," he replied, a bit sheepishly. "I couldn't lie."

"That is not a concern at present," I said. "Worry about that later. Right now I have some news for you. I guess you can tell that I'm out of surgery. We had a bit of a problem..."

"Jeremy's OK, isn't he? He better be OK," Mom almost threatened.

"He's OK, at the moment, but as we were working he started bleeding more, bleeding from places that should not have bled. His blood wasn't clotting. I did what I could do to control everything, but he's still not out of the woods and I'm not a hundred percent sure what the problem is."

"How is he now?" Dad asked, his voice filled with nothing but anxiety and worry.

"He's stable, blood pressure is normal, all his organs seem to be functioning. It looks like his body temperature dropped and blood doesn't clot well if you're cold. We're doing what we can to warm him and make sure there are no other clotting problems. I packed a bunch of surgical pads around the sites which were bleeding and that has controlled everything, at least for the moment. He will need to go back to surgery in about 48 hours to remove them. In the meantime we need to correct his temperature and any other abnormalities. And, hope he doesn't bleed anymore."

But, he did continue to bleed. Besides his low body temp, his coagulation studies were abnormal. Most likely all these physiologic abnormalities were intertwined. Blood clotting is a complicated series of events which starts with platelets plugging a hole in a blood vessel, followed by a cascade of enzymatic reactions which lead to a mature clot. Biochemistry teaches us that such reactions work best at normal body temperature. Thus, significant lowering of body temperature causes derangement of normal clotting. And, once a body starts oozing it tends to beget more oozing, sometimes leading to the flood I witnessed within Jeremy's belly. My decision to pack around the site of bleeding and stem the tide for the moment, I hoped, would buy time to correct the underlying problems.

It worked, at first. I checked his coagulation status. His PT was elevated at 22 and his PTT was 48. His platelets were OK at 110,000. The nurses were working on warming him with a heating blanket and warmed fluids. He was transfused two jumbo units of FFP, plasma which would replace the clotting factors which had been consumed.

Maybe he's out of the woods.

But, eight hours later, at four in the morning, his heart rate started to rise, his blood pressure dipped, and his hemoglobin dropped from 10 to 8. There were a few bright spots. His body temperature was normal and his PT was down to 17 and PTT was normal.

"Transfuse two units PRBC's and give another jumbo unit of FFP," I ordered. "I'll be in to see him."

What to do? What to do? There must be some blood vessel which continues to bleed. Should I operate again? I've already been there. Maybe, maybe there's a better alternative? Think…think. Yes, there is another alternative which might work. I hope Dr. L. is on call.

My plan was simple. Rather than dig through the injured liver looking for the source of bleeding, the problem would be approached from a different angle.

"I know you don't like to get up early, but I really need your help," I explained to Dr. L. I told him the whole story.

"Do you think you can do an arteriogram and embolize whatever hepatic artery is bleeding?" I finally requested.

"It might work," he concluded, "although I've never embolized for this type of injury before."

It was true. Angiography and embolization of arteries for trauma is commonplace these days, 25 years ago such a practice was sporadic.

I called Jeremy's Mom and Dad and explained his condition and the plan.

An hour later, he was wheeled down to the angiography suite.

I stretched out on the couch in the Doctor's Lounge.

Maybe I should go home and sleep for a couple of hours. With my luck I'll get called back as soon as I walk in the door.

I closed my eyes for a few minutes, until I was interrupted by a call from Dr. L.

"There was a tiny blush from a branch of the right hepatic artery. I did a subselective embolization of the right hepatic. I think he'll be better," Dr. L. reported.

"Thank you," was all I said.

6:30. I guess I'll make rounds and then check on Jeremy.

Jeremy did stabilize. His heart rate came down to 95, BP stayed around 110/60, he was awake and alert, talking, wanting to eat.

"Clear liquids for now and we need to take you back to surgery tomorrow to remove all those packs," I reminded him and his parents.

I scheduled the next procedure for the next day to be done around 4:00 p.m. Unfortunately, I was on call that day and had to deal with a perforated ulcer before tackling Jeremy. It was around 7:00 p.m. when the OR crew came to pick him up.

"I'll be out to talk to you as soon as I'm done," I reassured Mom and Dad and a multitude of other relatives and friends.

"Could you talk to another doctor on the phone" Mom asked.

Really, do I have to?

"Another relative?" I asked, a bit facetiously.

"It's Dr. Red Duke," she added.

"Oh, OK."

Dr. Red Duke was a local celebrity. He was a general surgeon at the Texas Medical Center, was regularly featured on local news shows where he would explain a variety of medical and surgical maladies and what to do about them. Outside of that, I really didn't know him.

"Hello, this is Dr. G."

"This is Dr. Red Duke," he answered in his thick Texas drawl. "Tell me what you're dealin' with thar, young fella."

I presented the case as succinctly as I could and he listened without interruption.

"Sounds like you've done a fine job, Doctor. My only advice is that when you remove those lap pads, soak them in peroxide first. If you do that, they won't stick and you won't stir up any new bleeding. Good Luck."

"Thank you, now. I think they're waiting for me."

I hung up and headed to the OR where they really were waiting on me.

"Sorry to keep you waiting," I explained, "but I had to get some advice from Dr. Duke."

"You mean Red Duke."

"Sho 'nuff," I answered in my best Texas accent. "The family called him. Now let's get this done with."

This return to OR was most uneventful. There was only a couple hundred cc's of old dark blood, the packs easily came out after soaking them with saline and there was no bleeding. The abdomen was washed out; I left a drain by the liver and closed him up.

Maybe I can get a full night's sleep.

No such luck. I was in bed by 10:00, but at 1:00 the phone rang.

"Jeremy is very short of breath. He's breathing at about 36 (normal 12-16), his oxygen saturation is 90% on 100% nonrebreather, heart rate is 120, BP is high at 150/95."

"I'll be in to see him."

I'm getting tired of this.

For the third night in a row I climbed out of bed and made the 20-minute drive to the hospital.

Jeremy was sitting upright in bed, his oxygen mask in place, breathing at a rate of about 28.

"What's going on, Jeremy?" I began. "Any pain?"

"Just feel winded, like I can't get enough air into my lungs."

His oxygen saturation was at 91%, heart rate was 120. BP and urine outputs were OK. His chest X-ray looked a bit congested and there were bilateral pleural effusions, which means fluid around his lungs.

"Do you think we need to intubate him, Dr. G?" the ICU nurse asked.

"Give him some Lasix, 40 mg, now. I'm going to talk to Pulmonary."

I called Dr. P. and told him the story, while Jeremy got the Lasix.

"Dr. P. will be in," I told the nurse, but I could already see improvement with the Lasix.

Jeremy put out about 4 liters of urine. His breathing calmed and he began a steady improvement. His bilirubin rose to about 6, possibly related to the embolization of his liver, but then came down to normal.

There was no more bleeding, no respiratory difficulty, he was soon up walking and eating and he went home about twelve days after the original injury.

The control of bleeding utilizing angiography and embolization was a technique I had used prior to Jeremy, primarily for bleeding secondary to pelvic fractures and bleeding from tumors which could not be accessed surgically. The technique now is more common, often being used for trauma to the spleen, as well as liver and the aforementioned pelvic fractures. It is a true life saver in those cases where the patient has an isolated injury to an organ which will tolerate the embolization.

The liver has a dual blood supply, receiving blood from the hepatic artery and the portal vein. In this case, embolization of the artery did the trick.

I saw Jeremy about four years later. He came to see me because he thought he had a hernia. He had given up riding in the rodeo and was working locally as an electrician. He did not have a hernia.

His Dad paid me ten dollars a month for a couple of years, determined to make up for the lack of insurance. I told my office staff to write off the balance and forgive the rest of his debt after about two years.

I stay away from horses, except for the occasional trips to the race track.

THE WRONG PLACE…

I was just walking down the hall, minding my own business, planning to make rounds on a few hospital patients, when I was spotted. One of the ER doctors was walking down the other end of the hall. We waved at each other and I went on my way. But, not for long.

"Call ER, stat," read the message which appeared 5 minutes later.

"Dr. Gelber, call ER," sounded overhead.

I'm not on call, at least I don't think I am.

"This is Dr. Gelber, I was paged," I said as the ER answered.

"This is Dr. A. I know you're not on call, but I saw you walking down the hall. I've got a lady here that needs a surgeon right away. She's 75, came in complaining of passing out, along with abdominal and back pain. I did a stat CT of her abdomen and she's got a 'leaking abdominal aortic aneurysm.' Can you come and see her?"

It's going to mess up my day. Well, maybe not. I guess I'm not terribly busy today.

"OK, I'll be there in a minute. Is she stable? Have you typed and crossed her?"

"Her BP is 90/50. She's had a liter of fluid."

"OK."

Ginny was 75, with a history of hypertension, COPD, and cigarette smoking. She was awake and talking when I saw her. Her abdomen was tender and there was a definite pulsatile mass, the typical finding when there is an abdominal aortic aneurysm.

CT of the abdomen/pelvis revealed fluid an infrarenal aneurysm surrounded by fluid, presumably blood, and normal iliac arteries.

"You're going to need surgery Ginny, or else you won't survive," I explained. "The major artery in your abdomen has weakened and now has burst. Half of the people who have ruptured aneurysms die suddenly and, of those who make it surgery, half survive. Do you understand?"

She nodded her head.

I've made that speech about a twenty times in my career, almost always those exact words. So far, no one has refused surgery. It is a fact of medicine that the mortality of untreated ruptured abdominal aortic aneurysm is 100%.

I called up to the OR.

"Hello, this is Dr. Gelber, y'all busy up there?" I asked a bit nonchalantly, I guess.

"Yes, what can I do for you?" asked Miss B., one of the surgical techs.

"Well, I've got this patient here in the ER with a ruptured abdominal aneurysm and she needs to come to surgery right away."

"You're kidding, right?" was Miss B's incredulous reply.

"No, she definitely has an aneurysm and it's definitely ruptured. I need to go right away."

"Oh, shit… I'll get right back to you."

And she hung up.

I called back immediately.

"This is not a 'wait and see, get to it when we can' situation. How long will it take you to get ready?" I asked, trying to convey the idea that this was an immediate, life threatening emergency.

"We'll be ready in twenty minutes."

"Good, she's signing her consent and she's typed and crossed, so you can send for her now."

I sat in the small Doctor's Lounge while the OR crew wheeled Ginny up to surgery.

Get in quick, get control either at the diaphragm or at the neck of the aneurysm. Be careful of the left renal vein and the duodenum. Looks like a straight graft will work, at least based on the CT Scan appearance. Oh, and don't make a hole in the vena cava or the duodenum.

Most of the time I don't sit and think about the dos and don'ts of an operation. Gallbladders, hernias, bowel resections are so ingrained that the potential pitfalls are dealt with almost by second nature.

Ruptured aortic aneurysms are different. Once the belly is opened the situation can deteriorate to chaos in seconds. Exsanguinating hemorrhage may occur before the aorta is even identified. The few moments before the operation begins are akin to a fighter psyching himself up before the big match.

Ginny was now on the OR table and I made the short walk down the hall from lounge to OR Five. As she went to sleep I washed my hands and we were ready to start.

I made a xiphoid to pubis incision and went to work. Fascia was divided, bowel was retracted, and I was greeted by the retroperitoneum obscured by blood. Dark hematoma surrounded the duodenum and caused the posterior peritoneum to bulge, pulsating with each heartbeat.

Get some sort of proximal control first. Start where you can at least see something, where it's safe. At least she still has a good blood pressure.

I put my hand up behind the left lobe of the liver, just below the diaphragm, and felt for the aorta. There was an NG tube in the esophagus and I pushed this structure to the left and quickly worked my hand down to the aorta and compressed it. Ginny's Blood pressure rose from 80 to 110.

"Do you have the aortic compressor?" I asked. I received a puzzled look. "It's a T-shaped thing that is used to push down and compress the aorta."

A light went on in the surgical tech's eyes and she reached to her back table.

"Is this it?"

"Yeah."

I took the compressor (I'm not sure if that is its proper name) and positioned it where my hand was and pushed down.

"Hold this here," I instructed my assistant.

I went to work on the aneurysm, opening the peritoneum over the aneurysm and adjacent to the duodenum, beginning to wade through the extensive hematoma which surrounded the aorta.

Don't injure the duodenum, don't injure the left renal vein, and do not injure the vena cava. Just find the aorta. Quickly, quickly.

I dug the duodenum from the swamp of clot and carefully divided the peritoneal attachments, moving up and to the right, of the presumed location of the aorta. I continued wading through the hematoma which brought me down to the aneurysm. I used my finger to dissect along the surface of the aneurysm, superiorly, hoping to find the normal aorta above the ballooning aorta.

There should be a hole in this aneurysm somewhere.

As soon as this thought popped into my head, I saw a stream of blood welling up from the posterior aspect of the left side of the aneurysm.

Need to work faster. There it is.

The aneurysm narrowed to normal caliber aorta. I continued dissecting with my finger around the neck of the aneurysm until I reached the vertebral body behind the aorta.

"Aortic clamp, please," I requested.

The surgical tech popped it into my hand and I slid it down around the aorta just above my fingers and closed it.

"Let up on that aortic occlude," I directed my assistant.

"Good, good, looks like we've got pretty good proximal control," I announced.

I half expected some cheering from the bleachers, but all I got was silence as we continued to work. It had taken ten minutes to gain proximal control of the aorta.

Next I began to dissect along the inferior aspect of the aneurysm, looking for the bifurcation of the aorta and the iliac arteries. Staying close to the aneurysm wall, I was rewarded with the inverted "Y" as the aorta divided into common iliac arteries.

At least the iliacs are not aneurysmal. Makes it a little easier.

Years ago, as a newly-minted attending surgeon, I had assisted one of the Chief Residents on what was supposed to be a ruptured aortic aneurysm. The problem with that case was that as soon as we opened the abdomen, it was obvious that the aneurysm was not ruptured. There was no question that the patient had an aneurysm, a huge one which also extended to the iliac and femoral arteries. I was left with a dilemma. Should I proceed with repairing the aneurysms, an operation which would have taken 5-6 hours in a patient who had presented in shock, only now it was apparent that the hypotension was due to a cause unrelated to his aneurysm? Or, stop the operation, close the patient and figure out why he was hypotensive. This complex clinical scenario was one of the few times I sought the opinion of one of my more seasoned colleagues. We both agreed that to proceed would be a death sentence for that patient, thus the aneurysm repair was aborted. It turned out that this patient had a combination of gastrointestinal bleeding and severe congestive heart failure. He recovered from the surgery, but died suddenly three weeks later. Perhaps his aneurysm ruptured at that later date?

But, back to Ginny.

I dissected each common iliac artery and clamped them. The bleeding from the aneurysm pretty much stopped.

Now it's time to start the operation.

Indeed, the aorta was controlled. The next step was to repair the aneurysm. I cut through the ballooned out anterior wall, opening the aorta. Old clot was scooped out. There was back bleeding from a number of lumbar arteries which arose from the back wall of the aneurysm. Each was sutured with 2-0 silk. There was vigorous back bleeding from the inferior mesenteric artery (IMA).

Great, I can ligate the IMA.

What the back bleeding meant was that there was adequate collateral circulation to the colon and ligation of the IMA should be safe. That is, ischemia of the left colon should not develop due to interruption of its blood supply.

With all the bleeding controlled the task was down to sewing in a graft. I measured the aorta at 20 mm, selected the appropriate graft and went to work. First the back wall of the proximal anastomosis, then the suture was run around until the two ends met anteriorly and were tied together. The graft was clamped and the moment of truth arrived. The clamp on the proximal aorta was released. I was rewarded with the graft filling with blood, pulsing, but not leaking.

Amazing. I did it right on the first try for once.

It was common to have to place a few reinforcing sutures if there was any bleeding from the anastomosis.

Next, the distal end of the graft was sewed into place. The clamps were taken off the iliacs, one at a time and flow was restored to the legs. There were pulses palpable in each iliac and femoral arteries.

Am I really done? It's only been an hour and twenty minutes.

"2-0 vicryl, please," I asked as I prepared to close the aneurysm over the graft.

Wait, where's that blood coming from?

Dark blood was now welling up from around the graft.

"Looks venous," I commented out loud to anyone that may have been paying attention.

I hope it's not the vena cava. More likely a small branch or lumbar vein.

Suction and more suction allowed me to see that the blood was coming from above the proximal part of the graft.

The left renal vein?

Not exactly. The blood was from a branch which was going to the left renal vein.

The ovarian vein.

I clipped it and the bleeding stopped.

"Irrigation and 2-0 Vicryl," I asked again.

This time I was able to close, first the aneurysm was closed over the newly placed graft and then the peritoneum, return the bowel to the abdomen, close the fascia and skin and be done with it. Two hours skin to skin.

Now comes the hard part.

Ginny was wheeled into the ICU and she looked pretty good. Her blood pressure was 105/60, heart rate was 90 and her oxygen saturation was 100%. There was some urine in the Foley bag and she had palpable pulses in her feet.

Maybe she'll just breeze through the post op period and be out of here in a week.

I just shouldn't allow myself to be so optimistic, because every time I have such fantasies my hopes and dreams are dashed.

As always I stayed around while Ginny was hooked up to all the monitors, ventilator, and everything else. Orders were written, the op note dictated, and her family was apprised of her condition and the findings at surgery.

After all the necessary post op chores were completed, I checked on her. Her blood pressure had dropped to 80/40.

"Give her a fluid bolus, 1000 cc Lactated ringers, and make sure her lab is sent. I need to see her H/H," I commanded, standing at the foot of the bed, directing the nurses like an admiral.

I checked her feet again. Even though her blood pressure was low and her legs were cool, I could feel her pedal pulses fairly easily.

I just need to fill her tank after the surgery.

Patients who undergo surgery for abdominal aortic aneurysms, particularly ruptured AAA's, will require large amounts of IV fluids and blood products after surgery. When the aorta is clamped, the distal vessels, that is those in the pelvis and lower abdomen constrict, arteries and veins. After the graft is in place and flow to the lower body is restored, these vessels will dilate over time. If the volume is not replaced, the blood pressure will drop.

I assumed this was the case with Ginny. Her H/H came back at 10/30, a little low but adequate. Her blood pressure came up with the IV fluids and I relaxed.

However, an hour later her blood pressure fell to 70. *Still needs more volume.*

I gave her another liter of fluid and a couple of units of Packed Red Blood Cells. She responded as expected and her blood pressure rose to 105/50. She was starting to wake up, opening her eyes and moving her arms and legs. Her urine output was low, about 40 cc since the surgery had ended.

This may not be good. Kidneys look like they are shutting down, BP is up and down. Everything suggests that she is dry. Maybe she's bleeding? If there was a real leak from her anastomosis, she'd be far more unstable or dead. Probably just a bit of oozing.

"Check her coags, PT/PTT, bleeding time and get another H/H," I continued to command from the foot of the bed.

Ginny's blood pressure dropped again, only now her EKG looked different, specifically she was displaying elevate ST segments, a finding suggesting she was having a myocardial infarction. I called her Cardiologist, Dr. M.

"Hello, John, I just finished operating on a patient of yours, Ginny S. She had a ruptured Triple A. Surgery went very smoothly, but she is not behaving herself. I think she's having an MI. ST segments are elevated, blood pressure is up and down," I reported. "EKG tech just arrived to do a twelve lead. Ruptured aneurysm and acute MI is a bad combination."

He voiced his agreement with my assessment and said he would be in to see her shortly.

That is what I call bad luck, MI on top of a ruptured aneurysm. Makes for a poor prognosis. So much for an uncomplicated post op course.

Her family was in the room now and I gave them the update on her condition. Dr. M arrived at that moment.

"Her best chance is to have a cath," he concluded, staring at the monitors.

Her blood pressure was around 90 systolic, but now her heart was having frequent premature beats and short runs of ventricular tachycardia.

"Do what you have to do, John. If she needs to be anticoagulated, go ahead, although it would be better if you can wait a few hours," I advised.

About an hour later, Ginny was wheeled down the hall to the cath lab, four hours after her surgery.

It's not fair for a body to have to survive two life threatening conditions in one day.

Ginny was in the cath lab for more than two hours. I managed to address three semi emergencies during this time. Finally a message came through from Dr. M.

"Three vessel disease, three stents placed."

I called him and got the full story. Thirty minutes later, Ginny was back in the ICU. She now had a Swan Ganz catheter in place.

The Swan Ganz catheter used to be a vital tool to assist in managing complicated, critically ill patients.

It is essentially a continuous right heart catheterization which allows for the measurement of pressures in the central veins and the pulmonary artery. A balloon on the end of the catheter, when inflated, occludes the pulmonary artery which allows a "wedge" pressure to be obtained. This is supposed to be a reflection of left heart pressure. Information gleaned from the S-G catheter is supposed to help with fluid management. The use of these catheters has diminished after a landmark study which showed that the measurements obtained from The S-G catheter were often misleading, which may have led to more harm than benefit to patient care and outcome.

Dr. M. had decided, justifiably, that Ginny would benefit from the monitoring and data gathered from the Swan Ganz. I was inclined to agree. A patient after surgery for a ruptured AAA usually requires large volumes of fluid, particularly in the early post op period. A patient with an acute MI has opposite needs. Cardiac function is likely impaired and too much fluid could easily send a patient into heart failure. Ginny's management would be very testy over the next few days. Her prognosis for survival also was very poor; she needed every break to weather this storm.

No urine output.

"No urine output," I repeated, out loud this time.

I called Dr. K., the Renal specialist.

It was 8 hours after the cardiac cath. She was on low dose Dopamine and was maintaining a blood pressure around 100, heart rate of 100 also.

Ruptured AAA, acute MI, of course renal failure and dialysis would be next. And in 48 hours it will be ARDS, then a trach, sepsis, probably ischemic bowel, if she makes it that far. One problem at a time for now, I hope.

Dr. K came and diagnosed Acute Tubular Necrosis. I placed a dialysis catheter and prepared to settle in for the long haul. Ginny began to stabilize after a day, at least her blood pressure stabilized at around 110/60. She required only low dose dopamine, but still no urine output. She was awake and following commands, which meant she was aware of the happenings around her.

Maybe, she'll turn the corner.

But, the next day her oxygen saturation dropped to 91%, despite increasing her inspired oxygen level from 50% to 70% and finally to 100%. At that level, she saturated at 95% and she stabilized again. My cautious optimism returned. Unfortunately, Ginny didn't agree. Her blood pressure dropped into the 80's and it became even more difficult to maintain her oxygenation.

We physicians were stuck. The only way to improve her oxygen saturation would be to add Positive End Expiratory Pressure or PEEP. Unfortunately, this has a side effect of decreasing the return of blood to the heart which leads to a drop in blood pressure. Ginny's Pulmonary and renal consultants spent the next few days balancing on a tightrope of low levels of PEEP mixed with a cocktail of pressor agents, which are infusions such as Dopamine and Levophed, medications which drive the heart as well as having an effect on blood vessels to augment cardiac output and help maintain adequate blood pressure. The ultimate goal is to maximize perfusion of Ginny's end organs: her brain, liver, muscle, skin and everything else.

And, it seemed to be working. She was awake and cognizant of her surroundings, able to follow commands. Her GI tract started working which allowed her to receive enteral feeding via an NG tube, instead of Total Parenteral Nutrition into a vein; the enteral route being much more physiologic with less potential for complications.

She smoldered along in the ICU for the next few days, not getting any worse, but not much better, either. The dance between pressor agents, PEEP and dialysis was choreographed to perfection. Her oxygenation gradually improved with saturations reaching 95%, while her blood pressure remained adequate, but still only rare drops of urine found their way into the Foley bag.

No more disasters, I hope. Just don't get worse and you should make it.

"She'll need a trach," Dr. P. advised. "I don't see her getting off the vent any time soon."

I was inclined to agree. Two days later, which was about nine days post op, we did the tracheostomy. A week later, little had changed. Every time we tried to drop her Dopamine or Levophed, her blood pressure fell into the 70's and 80's. We did manage to get her supplemental oxygen requirement down to 60% and eliminated the PEEP.

Baby steps are better than nothing.

But, something always has to happen.

"Ginny's fingers and toes are turning blue," the night nurse reported.

I was about to leave for rounds when her call came through. I changed my planned route so that I could see her first. Sure enough, her digits were cyanotic. I could feel her pulses and her arms and legs were warm.

"We need to get her off those pressors," I told the nurse. "Take that as an order," I added facetiously.

I also decided to anticoagulate her, hoping that the blood thinning effects of heparin would halt the progression of the impending gangrene.

I wish you would decide to get better, Ginny. This one step forward, two steps back, three steps to the side is frustrating for all of us, including you, I'm sure. You're smiling at me? Maybe you can read my thoughts.

And so it went, for a few more days, which dragged on to a couple of weeks. I think her heart found new strength as the pressors were weaned off. The tips of three fingers one each hand and nine of her toes developed gangrene.

Then, more than a month into her illness it came: a bit more urine. First it was 10 or 20 cc an hour, the 25, then 30 cc an hour. Her lungs improved and she was weaned off the ventilator.

She began to eat on her own, breathe on her own, and was fast reaching the point where she would be ready to get out of bed, maybe even take a few real baby steps.

A week later she was deemed ready to move to a skilled nursing unit, seven weeks after the initial insult.

I didn't see her for about two months. She walked into my office one afternoon.

"Thank you," she said, "thank you for saving my life."

"It's my job," I replied, "but, give yourself some credit. You are a fighter and that is as important as anything I did."

"I guess it wasn't my time," she added.

So, Ginny survived. Her successful outcome was a true team effort, as the combined skills of surgery, critical care, renal, cardiology, nurses, and technicians brought her back from the brink several times.

I saw the ER physician, Dr. A, about a month after I last saw Ginny. He asked about the ruptured AAA he had drafted me to attend to.

"Oh, Ginny?" I answered. "She did OK. She threw us a few curves, but she's OK."

I smiled to myself as I thought about my being in the wrong place at the right time.

MY NIGHT WITH PAULA

I don't think I'll ever forget that night. We were together for hours, standing and sitting near each other, hands mingling together as we kept at it, long and intense; endless. The minutes stretched into hours, but we would not give in to fatigue. Finally, I looked up and stared into her soft hazel eyes. I'm not sure what I was looking for: maybe some soft words of encouragement or some good thoughts. She seemed to sense my anxiety, my deep needs as I stared into those eyes. It wouldn't have taken much, maybe just a nod of her head, to keep me going. It seemed like an eternity, but then those eyes lit up and the light danced in them. Then I heard the words I'd been waiting for:

"Why don't you just cut the damned leg off?"

"Harrumph," was my reply and bent my head and went back to work, doing my best to salvage poor Melvin's leg.

Melvin was a retired mailman. He'd spent most of his life walking and the blocked artery prevented him from pursuing this favorite activity. He could barely go fifty feet when I first met him.

"The pain in my calf is just terrible, Doc," he reported. "I can't do anything anymore, Can't you help me?"

He went through the usual evaluation which revealed a fairly straightforward occlusion of the right superficial femoral artery with pretty normal arteries beyond the blockage. He still smoked cigarettes and had hypertension. In short, he was the typical vascular patient. I had advised him to give up smoking and he had cut back from two packs per day to half a pack; an improvement, but not the complete abstention I would have liked.

His symptoms warranted surgery and he underwent an uneventful right femoral-popliteal bypass, six months before Paula and I were to come together for our eventful night.

Melvin called my office complaining of severe pain in his leg the day before. A quick exam confirmed that his graft was occluded. Off to the hospital he went, a friendly Radiologist whisked him to the angio suite where catheters were inserted into his arteries and an attempt was made to dissolve the offending clot. Unfortunately, the thrombolysis didn't work. The catheter could not be properly positioned in the graft, and a day of infusing thrombolytic medication did nothing. Melvin's leg was still ischemic.

Surgery was the next option. A simple thrombectomy. Open up the groin run the Fogarty up and down a few times, close the artery, and be done in less than an hour. The best laid plans…

The whole affair did not begin well. I had been waiting for hours to begin the surgery. I called the OR at about 5:00 p.m. and asked Melissa, the head nurse on evenings, when I'd be able to start my case. Melvin's foot did have some circulation and he was not in any immediate danger of losing his it, but he was having considerable pain.

"Come on now," was Melissa's answer.

So, I made the short drive over to the hospital.

"You have to wait for Dr. so-and-so to finish," she announced after I arrived.

"But, you told me to come in now," I protested.

"I thought the other room would be done and anesthesia can only run one room," she replied.

This was a common Melissa *modus operandi*, that is tell me to come to do a case when it really wouldn't start for hours. After two or three of these charades, I learned not to come in unless they were definitely ready to start. But, for Melvin I waited and waited and waited. Almost three hours later, at about 8:00 p.m., we were ready to start. Initially, Martha was the surgical tech scrubbed on the case, but she had to leave at about 9:00, replaced by Paula. We had barely scratched the skin at that point.

The incision and initial dissection were unremarkable. There was the expected scarring, but the graft was easy to expose and the dissection of the scarred tissue surrounding the common, superficial, and profunda femoris arteries was not unusually difficult.

"This shouldn't take much longer," I said to Paula as she tied her gown and ambled up to the table. "Hopefully just run the Fogarty up and down and we'll be done."

"Good," was all she said.

The best laid plans of mice and men…

With the arteries exposed and controlled and everything in place, the real operation was ready to commence: give some heparin, clamp the arteries, open the graft, close to the anastamosis to the common femoral, and we're on our way.

As expected there was thrombus (clot) in the graft. The clot we could see was pulled out and then a #4 Fogarty catheter is passed, distally first, removing a long snake of maroon thrombus, a large amount first, and smaller amounts with each pass. There is a bit of resistance with the last pass, but no more clot is retrieved and we are rewarded by bright red blood filling up the graft, suggesting that the artery is open.

Now, the other way. The first pass restores some inflow, but not completely as the blood weakly squirts out, instead of the blast of blood under pressure one would expect from an unobstructed femoral artery. Two more passes and there is a sudden burst of bright red blood as normal inflow is restored.

Everything is going well, just close it up and we should be done.

I smile at Paula who is sitting across from me.

"We should be done soon," I comment.

"Good, because it's past my bedtime," she replies.

OK, sew up the graft with some 5-0 Prolene, open her up, good pulse here and down the graft. Check the foot: no pulse.

"Do you have a Doppler?" I inquire of the circulator.

"I've got it already," Paula states.

Always on top of things, that Paula.

I listen at the ankle. There is a weak regular pulse, audible, but not what I would expect if the graft was open. I listen over the graft and hear the short staccato of the pulse, like waves beating against a closed door.

"Something's not right," I say out loud to no one in particular. "Give me something to open up this graft again."

And, we start anew.

Pass the catheter, restore backbleeding, no pulse. OK, let's open up at the distal anastamosis. The old, healed wound at the distal thigh is incised and carried down to where the graft is encased in scar tissue. This scar is gingerly cut away, exposing the graft material which is cleaned down to the connection at the popliteal artery. There is a pulse in the graft, but none in the native artery.

Next step: clamp the graft and open the artery just above the distal anastamosis. The inflow is excellent and there is some backbleeding from the artery into the graft. Pass the catheter and it stops about ten centimeters into the graft. There must be some occlusion at that level. It's time to stop for a moment and look at the arteriogram.

The artery is open on this film. What's the problem? Must be a dissection of the artery.

"We may be here a while," I remark, once again to no one in particular. I look up at the clock, now reading 10:15 p.m.

"You may want to call in the call team," I remark. "We definitely will not be done by 11:00."

"That's me," Paula reports.

"I guess we're in this together," is all I can say.

I return to the patient and start to dissect more. Paula follows my every move, handing me scissors, clamp, pick-ups, right angle, vessel loop, whatever I need without my asking, anticipating my every need. I follow the graft down to the artery and begin to tease it away from scar tissue and delicate veins which entwine around the artery.

Careful, try not to tear anything.

A pool of dark blood wells up. Suction… suction some more. There's the culprit: a branch from one of the veins which surround the artery. Clip, clip, a bit more suction, then on with the fight. I'm reaching the limits of what I can dissect around the knee. The artery is diving deep behind the knee, a difficult place to expose. But, it looks like there is enough artery beyond the junction with the graft to work with.

Clamp. Clamp, cut and look inside the artery. There is no question that the artery is dissected, a bad thing in this case. What it means is that the lining of the artery, or intima, has lifted away from the muscular wall, creating a false passage. I'm left with two options: try to repair the dissected artery or bypass to a different spot, probably below the knee.

At this point I have to confess that I've never had much luck with repairing arterial dissections, although I keep trying. I don't know if it's my technique or if I underestimate the extent of damage. All I do know is that I've tried to do it over and over again, but I never learn, it never works and I always end up redoing the bypass at some point away from the damaged artery.

Even with the above disclaimer, I try to repair the artery. A number of interrupted 7-0 sutures tacking the back wall down, then close the artery and open the graft and, *voila*, a pulse appears in the artery.

Good, good, let's close up and be done with this case. But, it was not to be. After five minutes the pulse disappears and I'm back to square one. The clock now reads 1:30 a.m. I stare at the arteriogram and proceed.

Paula looks up at me from across the table, sighs, and hands me the scalpel. However, she's too slow anticipating my needs this time as I make the next incision below the knee using the cutting mode on the electrocautery, a sign that I am getting a little frustrated with the whole affair. Deeper and deeper into the leg, through fat, fascia, around muscle, more fat, more fascia until a bundle of veins is exposed. I perform a little more careful dissection and finally identify the popliteal artery below the knee, a hard pipe of calcified artery that, although appearing to be adequate on the X-Ray, will not serve my purposes, because the severe calcification would make it impossible to sew.

Maybe a bit more proximal?

Dissecting up a bit exposes more of the same. Now what? It's at this point Paula offers her words of encouragement.

"Why don't you just cut the damn leg off?"

It's now getting close to 3:00 a.m. and I'm not much better off than when we started. One last effort: bypass farther down the leg, to the anterior tibial artery, which looks good on the arteriogram and runs all the way into the foot.

At this point I recall a case I scrubbed on as a resident. I was helping one of the vascular surgeons do a similar case. This particular surgeon was one I considered to be of marginal skill at best. He had filleted the leg open in the groin, thigh, proximal leg, and was about to go to the ankle when I asked:

"Do you think this will work?"

Surprisingly, he didn't become angry or command me to leave the OR suite, much to my dismay. He just shrugged and replied that sometimes, in Vascular Surgery, you do what you have to do, because the alternative is loss of limb or life.

Paula and I embarked on the next stage of our journey as I began to expose the anterior tibial artery. The artery was small as expected, but appeared adequate for my purposes. I harvested a segment of saphenous vein from the groin and thigh, long enough to run from the graft in the thigh to the mid-calf. Next I opened the artery, greeted by some back bleeding. I embarked on the first anastomosis, vein to artery, with the vein reversed to avoid the problem of its valves. Next the vein was tunneled from the anterolateral leg to the medial thigh and then the next anastomosis was done, graft to vein.

And, the moment of truth, the clamps are removed and… nothing. No pulse in the new vein graft. I examine the graft in the groin, where there is a pulse and in the thigh, where there isn't.

Maybe, it's something simple, just some thrombus in the graft. The way this case is going there are probably gremlins inside the graft.

From the graft in the thigh I pass a Fogarty catheter proximally and distally and, thankfully, some clot is removed from the proximal graft. Now there is excellent inflow. The graft flushes easily with no resistance. I suture the graft closed and, crossing my fingers and toes, open it up to allow flow. To my, and Paula's, great relief there is a good pulse in the graft and in the artery beyond the graft.

It's now 8:00 a.m.

All that remains is to make sure there is no bleeding and close it up. Brian, Paula's relief, comes in and offers to take her place. To her credit, she volunteers to stay and finish what she has started. We put the last dressing on at about 9:00 a.m. We both leave for a much needed bathroom break, after which I sit down to the tedium of writing orders and dictating the marathon operative note.

Melvin recovered uneventfully. His graft remained patent for about eight months and then re-occluded. This time it was reopened by our Interventional Radiologist. It occluded again sometime later and he learned to live with the pain for a while. Eventually, he had to undergo a below knee amputation.

He underscores what one of my teachers told me years ago.

"All vascular surgery is palliative. What we do staves off the inevitable."

In medical school I worked with a resident who put it more bluntly:

"Vascular surgery patients don't get older, they just get shorter."

As I think about these words now, it strikes me that what he said can be applied to all of medicine. What we doctors do is purely palliative. The end result is the same for everyone and the best a physician can do is put off, for a time, the inevitable.

I did see Paula before she left that morning; both of us were exhausted, completely and totally spent, but also quietly satisfied after the night's affair. She has continued to assist me over the years, now as a Licensed First Assistant. She remains one of the best assistants, perhaps because she understands the way I operate better than most, one of the fruits of our long, arduous night together.

.

IMPOSSIBLE

"*First do no harm…*" Hippocratic Oath

What should a surgeon do with an impossible case? For the first time in my career I asked myself that question. Over the years, I've had more than my share of difficult cases. I've had patients with life threatening conditions whom I wished I could offer more than to just shake my head and speak empty words of encouragement. They stare back at me and I see their eyes full of hope. How many times have been forced to say: "I'm sorry, there's nothing I can do that will make you better, or cure you, or ease your pain."

I hate moments like those.

A patient comes to me with cancer of the stomach. Major surgery is scheduled. All the preoperative testing indicates that there is a good chance for the surgery to be curative. An incision is made and the abdomen is explored. My heart sinks with the first glance. Grayish white nodules stud the abdomen. The normal yellow fat of my trusted friend, the omentum, is caked with an ugly gray mass of cancer, despite the preop CT Scan that was reported as "no evidence of metastatic disease." Nothing can be done. "Maybe chemotherapy will shrink the tumor," I say, although I know that this cancer rarely responds. The cancer was there before the operation. The surgery offered hope and no harm was done. And, after all this, the patient thanks me. Irony.

Another patient comes with pain in his legs and black patches on his feet. He smokes two packs of cigarettes a day, has been hypertensive for years, and sporadically takes his medication. My exam reveals areas of dry (not infected) gangrene on his feet, bluish discoloration of his toes, and no pulses can be felt in the groins or feet. The patient is sent off for a battery of tests which confirm my suspicions. All of his major arteries from just below the aorta and throughout his legs are occluded. In this case there is no reason to try to do any surgery. Any operation will surely fail and probably leave the patient worse than he is now.

The two cases above were difficult, no question. But they were handled in the best way possible and in neither case was the patient harmed; Hippocrates fulfilled. Difficult, but not impossible.

But, there was Lucia, a thirty-seven-year-old lady who had been in federal prison for three years; the reason for her incarceration never revealed. She had previous surgery performed in Mexico, one for Crohn's disease, the other for carcinoma of the colon. Details of these surgeries were unavailable. During her three years in prison she had been on and off Total Parenteral Nutrition, which is receiving all of one's nutrition through an IV, and had required nasogastric tube placement for bowel obstructions on a regular basis. Her prison time reached its end while she was in the prison hospital at which time her TPN was abruptly stopped and she was discharged from the prison with instructions to go to the hospital right away.

Of course, she did not choose to go to a hospital close to the prison. No, she decided to travel 250 miles and show up in the ER where I happened to be on call. The ER workup demonstrated a definite small bowel obstruction characterized by dilated proximal bowel and a paucity of air in the colon. She reported no passage of stool or flatus for three weeks, hallmarks of a complete intestinal obstruction. CT Scan revealed some sort of mass surrounding and encasing her small bowel and possibly a portion of her colon.

Lucia was admitted to the hospital. A biopsy of the mass seen on CT revealed only inflammation, no cancer. But, her obstruction persisted.

Why not? As she recounted: "I've been in and out of the prison hospital almost every week for three years."

From my perspective there was no choice. After four days in the hospital without improvement, I bit the bullet and brought her to surgery to embark on what I presumed would be a long difficult case. I never bargained for the impossible.

Her abdomen was marked by a wide scar running from xiphoid to pubis which meant that I was likely to find adhesions (scar tissue) along the entire length of her abdomen and that I should not anticipate finding any relatively easy spot, free from adhesions, to enter the peritoneal cavity.

Start with the simple things first.

The wide scar was excised which carried me into the subcutaneous tissue, usually marked by yellow fat. Hers was filled with fat and grayish white scar. Gingerly I dug deeper, through the scar to the expected fascia, the fibrous tissue which surrounds our muscles and provides the strength we needed to hold our abdomen together.

Carefully, oh so carefully, the fascia was incised, separating as it is divided. I am greeted by bowel, intact and pink.

Maybe this won't be as complicated as I'd feared.

Wrong, wrong, wrong. I teased the bowel away from the undersurface of the abdominal wall and what should have been peritoneum, the thin membrane which lines and surrounds our abdominal viscera.

Be very cautious, gentle, not too much tension or traction.

No good, the distinctive flower of bowel mucosa stared back at me, indicating a hole in the bowel, as my preop worries were realized, forcing me to settle in for what was sure to be a very long process. The hole in the bowel meant I was committed. There would be no backing out now. I suppose I could have just repaired the hole, but such a repair without freeing the bowel from all the adhesions would almost certainly break down resulting in a fistula. So, it was onward with the fight, diving further into the morass of fused bowels and adhesions. Lucia's and my troubles had barely started. Very gradually I managed to separate the abdominal wall from the underlying viscera. In the process I discover there was no "peritoneal cavity," only a solid mass of congealed intestine.

There must be one place where the bowel can be freed in a safe manner. Aha, this looks promising.

It turned out that it was and it wasn't. I was able to free that particular loop, but it was transverse colon, which does nothing to help me cure her small bowel obstruction.

Maybe here? No, just more colon.

The bowel in the middle was definitely small bowel and from its collapsed appearance and the CT Scan images, it was probably beyond the point of obstruction.

Maybe if I start with these dense adhesions?

No luck. Every attempt to pry even a centimeter loose threatened irreparable damage. At this point I also realized that she did not have much small bowel. She wasn't sure exactly what surgery she'd had before, but it appeared to me that she only had about three feet of small intestine and could not afford to lose anymore.

Try somewhere else. Maybe find the most proximal small bowel.

I gingerly attacked the left upper quadrant and was rewarded with some definitely dilated bowel. A little more dissection confirmed that it was small bowel.

At least I should be proximal to the point of obstruction.

Unfortunately, despite my cautious zeal, I made another hole in the small bowel. I toiled onward, gradually delineating the entire colon.

I was now left with the colon, which was completely free from scar tissue, a loop of dilated bowel, probably jejunum just beyond the Ligament of Trietz, (which marks the beginning of the small bowel beyond the duodenum) and then a solid mass of small bowel which was frozen together as if someone had embedded it in concrete.

I'm stuck.

If I tried to pry apart the remaining small bowel I would have caused such damage that the majority of her small bowel would have been unsalvageable, which would then require its resection and would have left her with almost no small bowel. If I just closed the holes I'd already made I maybe could back off, but she would still be obstructed and the closures would likely to leak. And she would have a fistula which would never heal.

Impossible.

I was now faced with a situation I'd never faced before. Over the years I've been in some very difficult abdomens, spent hours and hours teasing apart fused and fibrotic intestines. But I've always managed to get it all unstuck. Sometimes resection of irreparably damaged small bowel was necessary, most of the time only a few sutures to repair partial thickness tears were needed. But, now I was facing a new and, I hoped, unique situation. My instinct told me to stop, close the holes, and treat her with bowel decompression and time to see if she would resolve the obstruction without needing further intervention. My head told me this would leave her on TPN and with an NG tube forever.

Should I forge ahead, chisel away the concrete and pick up the pieces later, running the risk that irreparable damage could be done, which would be a death sentence? Maybe there's something else to do.

I knew that the loop of small bowel that I had freed from adhesions was dilated which meant it was proximal to the point of obstruction. The bowel in the mid-abdomen was collapsed and, thus, was beyond the obstruction.

What to do? Maybe a bit of probing will help. That's what doctors are supposed to do best.

I stuck my finger into the hole in the dilated bowel and felt downstream.

Yes, there was a definite tight stricture, a narrowed area which is most likely responsible for the obstruction. But how to fix it? My finger told me that the stricture was fairly short, less than two centimeters.

"GIA stapler, please," I asked.

The GIA is a device which places parallel rows of staples and cuts the tissue in between, closing off where the staples are fired, while opening in between. GIA stands for gastrointestinal anastamoser, or something like that.

I passed one side of the stapler through the stricture and left the other part of the stapler on the obstructed side, this all being done through the hole I previously made in the dilated bowel. Once I was sure everything was positioned properly I fired the stapler, performing a procedure which is properly termed a "stricturoplasty." Looking inside the bowel I saw that each staple line was in its proper location and there was no bleeding. I felt the area of the stricture and it was gone, the bowel now was wide open.

Success, I hope.

Now it was just a matter of closing the holes I'd made.

I'll keep my fingers, and toes, crossed, and hope that everything will heal.

I finished this impossible ordeal in about three hours. Now it was wait and see.

Have I relived her obstruction? Will she heal the "stricturoplasty"? Will she heal the intestinal closures? Will she ever be able to eat normally?

There was plenty to worry about; everything about this case had been a compromise and was far from ideal. Normally, I would have taken down all the adhesions, doing my best to be sure there were no unseen points of obstruction. Also, our bowels are not passive conduits. They are muscular tubes constantly contracting and moving. Repairing holes in bowels which are encased in adhesions allows for increased tension on the closure and, subsequently, increased risk of breakdown and development of a fistula. A fistula is an abnormal communication between two structures, such as bowel to bowel, or bowel to skin.

I've been toiling away at surgery for almost thirty years and this is the first time I ever found myself in such a difficult situation; a situation without a good solution, only compromises and guesses. Maybe I've been lucky, maybe it's been good planning, but I cannot recall any other case where there were no good intraoperative options, where it was impossible to back off and look for an alternative treatment, while going forward threatened to create bigger problems.

I suppose this case really did have options, but none of them was particularly satisfying. Even my final solution was fraught with danger, running the risk that she may still be obstructed with a high likelihood she would develop a fistula; it all boiled down to wait and see.

"To cut is to cure" goes the old saying, but for Lucia I'm not so sure. In retrospect her troubles started years before I ever saw her and my part in her care was only the end product of her disease process and previous treatment. Even so, the case leaves me with the feeling I could have done better.

Lucia had a stormy postoperative course. She did develop multiple fistulas and breakdown of the abdominal wound. Over the course of three months the fistulas and wound closed and she was able to eat small amounts. She still needed TPN, but she was able to go home. She was supposed to see me in my office about two weeks after her discharge, but she never appeared. Attempts to call her were greeted with the message that her phone had been disconnected.

But, eventually I learned her fate. She had been home for about ten days when she had a seizure. She was brought to the hospital closer to her home, but she arrested shortly after she arrived and expired.

She was only thirty four.

LUQECTOMY

Kerry was twenty-eight years old. He showed up in the ER one night complaining of upper abdominal pain which started suddenly that day. The Emergency physician did the usual workup and found two things which led to an urgent call: a large intrabdominal mass and free intraperitoneal air.

The large mass was not necessarily an emergency, but "free air," that is, air outside its usual place inside the bowel, almost always represents a surgical emergency; a perforation somewhere along the long snaking tube sometimes referred to as the "alimentary canal."

It was about midnight and I jumped, well, more likely slowly crawled, out of bed and made my way to the hospital.

Kerry had wispy brown hair which was coupled with a receding hairline. He made his living playing the guitar. He told me gigs came and went, but he managed to scrape by. He reported vague discomfort for about three months and weight loss of almost thirty pounds. He said he was able to eat, but often didn't feel hungry.

He was thin, almost cachectic, with pale skin, and his face betrayed a fear that I could tell was permeating his body and soul. The most significant finding on exam was diffuse abdominal tenderness with signs of peritonitis, just what one would expect from a perforated hollow viscus.

His abdominal CT scan demonstrated a large mass in the left upper quadrant of the abdomen, in the area of the left transverse colon, stomach, pancreas, spleen, left adrenal gland and left kidney. There was obvious free air and fluid.

No choice, he needs to go to surgery.

I explained the findings and the proposed surgery to him, wrote orders, called the OR crew, and then went to the physicians lounge to wait. The usual hour spent waiting for the team is something I've now figured out how to avoid. But, back in the old days, twenty years ago, I always came to see the patient first before deciding if emergency surgery was necessary, be it a simple case of acute appendicitis or a perforated colon with septic shock. This always afforded me an hour or so to meditate on the upcoming procedure or, more often, watch remnants of whatever old B movie happened to be on late night television.

Before starting Kerry's surgery, I spent the time considering what I was going to find inside of him. Free air suggested that the primary pathology was either in the colon or the stomach. The CT Scan suggested I be prepared to remove parts of the colon, stomach, pancreas, and spleen, a Left Upper Quadrantectomy, as I'd called it in the past.

I was sure he had a cancer of some sort, unusual and sad in someone so young. The tenants of cancer surgery dictate that it is best to remove the offending tumor *en bloc*, which means removing it all in one piece, preferably with a margin of normal tissue, something which is often not possible.

After my hour of contemplation, the nurse, tech, and Anesthesiologist were ready. Kerry was wheeled into the room and moved himself over to the OR table. I

couldn't help but notice the look in his eyes as he scooted from stretcher to OR table. It reminded me of looks
I'd seen in movies; seen on the faces of actors who are
made to walk up steps to the gallows or to the front of
a firing squad; a look of impending doom. I gave him
what I hoped was a reassuring smile as he positioned
himself in the middle of the narrow table. He did his
best to remain still as EKG leads, pneumatic compression stockings, and pulse oximeter were placed on the
appropriate parts of his body.

The steady, almost monotone voice of the anesthesiologist began:

"…take a deep breath, you may feel some burning
in your arm, you'll be asleep before…"

And Kerry was out.

Prep and drape, throw off the Bovie and suction,
and we're off.

I made a generous midline incision and soon entered his abdomen, neatly, exactly through the center,
to be greeted by a big ugly tumor. There was some thin
serous fluid and inflammation around the tumor which
was in closest proximity to the left side of transverse colon. I could see the hole where the tumor had perforated
into the omentum and observed only a small amount of
fecal contamination.

Good.

I gingerly moved the tumor, back and forth, up and
down. It was mobile. I've done cases in the past where
moving the tumor back and forth caused the whole patient to move, suggesting fixation of the tumor to vital
retroperitoneal structures, which means it is almost
surely unresectable and probably incurable.

It's time to do some work. First the colon.

I start on the left side, dividing the left colon's attachments up to its sharply angled turn at the splenic flexure, as well as dissecting the omentum free. Then, from the right. Here I start at the colon's beginning, the cecum. The appendix was stuck down in the pelvis. I free it up and notice it looks a little inflamed.

Appendicitis on top of everything else.

All along the right side of the abdomen I work, freeing the right colon up to the hepatic flexure and the proximal transverse colon, grateful that it easily lifted off the duodenum, that the tumor did not involve this part of the bowel.

No emergency Whipple tonight.

The right side of the omentum also was liberated, to be removed with the tumor. Now I started to surround the tumor. The back wall and greater curvature of the stomach were adherent to the mass, but this was limited to the most inferior portion. The vessels feeding this portion of the stomach were identified and divided, the stomach was then divided with a large stapler and the uninvolved portion of the stomach retracted away and out of sight.

One organ out of my way. What's next?

The colon needs to go now. His right colon is pretty short.

If I resect only the transverse colon, I'm not sure about the blood supply to the remaining segment on the right.

I decided to remove the complete right and transverse colon all the way to the proximal descending colon. This would allow for an anastomosis between the small bowel and descending colon, which should heal without problem, rather than a colon to colon connection in unprepped bowel. It was time for more staplers. GIA across the terminal ileum (last part of small bowel before the colon starts), again across the descending colon just beyond the splenic flexure.

I'm really zeroing in on this nasty beast now.

It became apparent that the tumor also involved the distal pancreas.

Maybe I can separate the two structures? No luck. The pancreas and the spleen will need to go.

This actually didn't take very long. Kerry was very thin and the border of the pancreas was easy to see, as were the splenic artery and vein. Dissection began along the inferior border of the pancreas until I reached an area at the neck of the pancreas which was uninvolved by tumor. The large splenic artery and vein were dissected free, clamped, and divided and ligated. The neck of the pancreas was divided using the GIA stapler and the pancreatic duct was also separately sutured. Finally, the vessels remaining which entered the spleen were divided and the specimen was removed *en bloc* as one giant mass of tissue composed of the omentum, right and transverse colon, greater curvature of stomach, tail of the pancreas and spleen.

Thus, I have completed the operation I have dubbed "Left Upper Quadrantectomy." This was really only a partial LUQectomy, as I was able to leave the left kidney and adrenal gland behind.

After removing this massive tumor I was left with the task of putting everything back together. In this case this it meant only a single anastomosis, small bowel to colon. I did leave a drain, just in case, and finished the entire procedure in just under two hours. Kerry was safely deposited in the recovery room and I manage to get home by about 4:30 a.m. to grab a couple of hours rest before the new day started.

Kerry had an uneventful postoperative course, out of the hospital in eight days. His tumor was adenocarcinoma of the colon, which is the most common type of colon cancer, but still unusual in someone so young. The size and presence of perforation put the cancer at a later stage. He was treated with chemotherapy and I wish I could report that he responded well and lived many years, but this was not the case. Even the best operation sometimes cannot overcome a cancer's inherent biology. Kerry's cancer recurred and he passed away eighteen months after his emergency operation. Still, he was remarkably pain free during this time and was able to play his guitar up to the end.

The LUQectomy is an operation I do about once a year, most times planned, but sometimes emergent.

Mary was a case similar to Kerry, only her tumor arose from the pancreas and presented with bleeding and perforation. She also had middle of the night, emergency surgery, the night cap to a day that included eight other scheduled and emergency cases.

I've attacked the left upper quadrant for tumors arising from stomach, colon, pancreas, adrenal gland, and retroperitoneum. The pathology may vary, but the approach is almost always the same. Find a plane free of cancer and isolate the tumor; try to get a margin of normal tissue. Always be aware of what can be safely removed and what needs to stay behind. Know where the major blood vessels are and treat them with the proper respect.

It is truly amazing how much can be removed with little or no subsequent physiologic impairment. Large portions of the pancreas can be removed, yet the patient never develops diabetes or malabsorption. All of the stomach could be removed and rebuilt with small bowel. But the patient continues to eat, although some weight would probably be lost. Portions of the colon are removed frequently for a variety of reasons, but very well tolerated. The body has two kidneys and two adrenal glands and can easily compensate for loss of one. The spleen is removed routinely for trauma or disease, yet is often barely missed.

Thus, the LUQectomy demonstrates the remarkable, incredible resiliency of the human body. Despite invasion by cancer and serving as a battlefield for the surgeon's war against this malignant enemy, despite the removal of large parts of vital organs, we are able to persevere. Truly amazing.

BEDSIDE

Today I thought about sitting at the bedside of pa-tients. I wasn't thinking about *sitting*, rather than standing, in the consultation room when first meeting new patients, which always a good practice as it sends the patient the message that you care enough about them that you are willing to spend the time to *sit* and listen to them. Rather, it was sitting at the bedside of the very sick patient; being right there to tend to their needs should an urgent situation or sudden change develop.

"That's the nurse's job," one may say, and in a sense that would be correct. But, sometimes a doctor needs to be present. As a medical student I was sheltered from sitting with the sickest patients. I did see some sick pa-tients as a medical student, but, always from a distance, on rounds, or as part of a presentation. I was never al-lowed to truly get involved in their minute-to-minute care. My first bedside experience with a really sick pa-tient was during the first month of surgical internship.

One night on call I was called to the ER for a pa-tient who had been stabbed in the upper abdomen. The patient was unstable, with severe tachycardia, hypoten-sion, and a stab wound between the xiphoid process of his sternum and his umbilicus. He was whisked away to the OR in short order, where the Chief resident and second-year resident spent the better part of the evening battling to keep this unfortunate patient, Jose, alive. He had suffered injuries to the stomach, colon, superior mesenteric artery, and vein and duodenum. I wasn't with them in surgery, but I did receive a call at about 1:00 a.m. to come to the ICU. They had just brought Mr. Gonzales from surgery and it was now my job to sit with him and attend to his needs.

I immediately noted the drains coming out of his abdomen, filling up with bright red blood.

"Just transfuse him as needed," were all the instructions I was given.

I gave him a quick once over. His pupils were nonreactive, his extremities were cold, there was no urine forthcoming from the Foley and three abdominal drains were already filled with blood. His heart rate was 130 and BP 75/35. I pulled up a chair, but didn't sit. For the next four hours the nurse and I pumped blood and plasma and platelets and cryoprecipitate and more blood into poor Jose. As fast as we pumped it in, it ran out: through the drains, through his mouth, through his endotracheal tube, from everywhere. It was my first encounter with a severe coagulaopathy. He was cold, he had already received massive volumes of transfusions and his blood would not clot.

Finally, shortly after five am, I called the Chief resident and asked this question:

"How long do you want me to do this?"

I explained the situation and told him that Jose had been transfused over two hundred units of blood products and we were still at square one. I knew I was just a lowly intern, but I gave my opinion anyway.

"I think it's hopeless."

My Chief agreed and we stopped. Jose died about one hour later from his lethal injury, never having regained consciousness or any but the faintest signs of life.

Jose was one of the most desperate and intense bedside vigils I've sat through over my many years in practice; there have been many more.

I've written about some in my books, *Behind the Mask* and *Under the Drape*. Chapters in those books recount my experience with one unnamed patient who had a stormy immediate post op course after an elective aortic aneurysm repair and with Gerald, who experienced one complication after another and required multiple operations, surviving the worst case of ARDS (Adult Respiratory Distress Syndrome) I've ever seen.

These examples demonstrate that a sick patient often requires constant attention. It has been my practice to stay with my very sick patients during the immediate postoperative period until I'm sure they are stable. Most of the time this is a short vigil, sometimes only a brief visit in the Recovery Room or ICU, while at other times I will stand at the foot of the bed, staring at the monitors and foley bag, waiting and hoping and praying for the blood pressure to rise or the urine to start flowing or the pulse oximeter to begin displaying a true waveform, while trying to decide if I've forgotten something important or if something else needs to be done. Each physiologic indicator tells me the same thing. When they are all good it means that the patient is perfusing vital organs adequately, but when one or more are bad then the whole patient is bad.

Dora was such a patient. She was old, almost ninety. She had lived in the county run nursing home for longer than she could recall. She came one evening with a very distended abdomen, obstipation and vomiting. She told me her belly had been hurting for three days. In the course of my evaluation I asked her how old she was.

She answered, "Older than dirt, but a little wiser."

158 | *Amazing Days, Endless Nights*

Her workup suggested a cecal volvulus with perforation. This means that the right side of her colon had become twisted, then blew up like a balloon and finally popped, causing peritonitis, a very serious, life threatening condition. She arrived in surgery at about ten o'clock at night and underwent a right colon resection and ileostomy. This means the right side of her colon was removed and then the end was brought out to the abdominal wall where it would empty into a bag, like a colostomy except involving the small bowel rather than the large bowel. The reason the surgery is done this way is that in a very sick patient healing is of major concern and reconnecting (anastamosing) the two ends of the bowel although initially successful, may fall apart after ten days due to poor healing. This would put poor Dora back at square one.

Surgery finished around midnight. I stayed around in the ICU while she woke up. Her blood pressure hovered in the 70/30 range and her urine output was minimal. I was in and out of the ICU, ordering fluid boluses, anxiously awaited lab reports, watching the Foley bag, trying to wish a few drops of urine into the tubing.

Dora lay still in her bed, although she did open her eyes after a while. Her post op CBC came back and the hemoglobin was higher than it had been pre-operatively, even though she had not been transfused any blood. I checked again. Sure enough, her preop hemoglobin/hematocrit was 11.1/33.3 and now it was 11.6/35.0. These numbers told me two things. First, it was unlikely that she was bleeding and second, that she was hypovolemic. I drew these conclusions because bleeding will cause the hemoglobin level to fall. This fall may not always be immediately apparent, but in a patient like Dora, who had already received large volumes of IV fluids, bleeding of any significance would almost surely cause the hemoglobin level to fall.

The fact that she was hypovolemic can be concluded because the rise in hemoglobin suggests *hemoconcentration,* a long word which means she had lost fluid from her blood stream or intravascular space into the surrounding tissues, the extravascular space. Think of the blood vessels as a sieve. Fill the sieve with marbles and water. Before pouring the mixture into the sieve the combined volume of marbles and water may be one quart, with 50% of the volume marbles and 50% water. The marble level can be considered to be 50%. But, when you pour the mixture into the sieve, the water leaks out and the marble level becomes 100%. The hematocrit level is akin to the marbles, that is it is the percentage of blood volume made up by red blood cells. The fact that it has gone up suggests that fluid has been lost from the intravascular space (bloodstream) into the extravascular space. The bottom line was that she needed more intravenous fluid to fill up her tank, that is, the intravascular space.

I stayed at her bedside for a bit more than two hours, until I was sure she was stable, then disappeared for a few hours of sleep before the next day's trials began. Dora, after the first few rocky hours, perked up and sailed through her postoperative period like a twenty year old. I was able to do surgery to reverse her ileostomy about three months later.

Two years later I was called to see and elderly lady with a distended abdomen. Small bowel obstruction was suspected. I went to the ER and found a very old patient with a very distended abdomen.

I asked her how old she was and she answered, "Old than dirt, but a little wiser."

"Dora, how nice to see you again," I answered. "I wish we could meet under different circumstances sometime, however."

She agreed. Her X-Rays suggested she had a small bowel obstruction and lab tests were worrisome for ischemic or gangrenous bowel. Therefore, at about eleven o'clock that night she went back to surgery where I lysed adhesions, resected an ugly segment of gangrenous bowel and settled down at her bedside and repeated the events of two and half years before.

Once again, after a suffering through a few hours where her condition was touch and go, she stabilized and made an uneventful recovery. I didn't have the pleasure of seeing her again and I don't know at what age she finally passed away, but I hope I gave a few more years of quality life.

I still make it a habit of staying around until my patients are stable after major surgery, particularly when the patient has a life threatening condition like those suffered by Dora and Jose. I don't seem to have to do it as often as I used to. I credit this to improved intraoperative care by anesthesia, better preoperative preparation and, maybe a bit of fortune which has allowed me to avoid operating on extremely ill patients in the middle of the night.

One question does remain.

Have I ever sat at a patient's bedside just to sit with them?

What I mean is have I ever had a patient who I had grown close enough to and who was so ill that I wanted to stay with them just out of concern and worry over their condition? Even if there was nothing I could do?

I actually thought about this before I even began writing this article about being at the bedside and then, ironically, it came to the forefront during a recent conversation, which was held in the operating room while removing a nasty appendix. The anesthesiologist and circulating nurse asked me just that question. Apparently the topic had come up during the day and they wanted my input.

I thought for a while and I couldn't come to a definite answer.

I have had innumerable patients over the years in whom I have a taken a personal interest in their care. Most often these were very sick ICU patients who needed very close attention as their condition had the potential to rapidly deteriorate. Patients like Albert who was admitted with a Neurosurgical condition, but developed sepsis from an intraabdominal source, requiring emergency surgery, and Doris, a victim of a motor vehicle accident who had a missed colon injury and came to our ICU with severe sepsis, or John who also came to the ICU after inadequate treatment for a perforated colon.

These and so many other patients have received my utmost, careful attention to help them through the most critical parts of what were often very complicated illnesses. I never, however, developed a truly personal relationship with any of these patients. I only saw them in a professional sense during their illness and once or twice after they had recovered. I never went out with them for a drink or to play golf. I guess I have taken the medical school teaching to heart: Maintain a detached concern.

The acute nature of surgical diseases, particularly general surgical conditions, rarely allows the development of a close relationship prior to a surgical intervention. Even those patients with cancer who are scheduled to undergo surgery are seen only once or twice before their operations. I care a great deal about my patients from a professional perspective. But, I see my task as one of helping them through the most serious part of an illness or injury; to get them healthy enough to return to their lives apart from being sick.

That is the job of a surgeon.

Perhaps, however, I am missing something?

BIG BLUE

I had a brief encounter with Big Blue today. I was doing a fairly routine laparoscopic hiatal hernia repair when it appeared, staring me straight in the face. It wasn't lurking around the corner or hiding behind another structure, it was right there, only millimeters away from the area in need of repair. Such are the pitfalls and dangers we intrepid surgeons face on a daily basis.

Big Blue is better known as the Inferior Vena Cava, the largest vein in the human body. This monster's function is to receive deoxygenated blood from most of the veins below the diaphragm and return it to the heart for processing, which means dumping unwanted carbon dioxide in the lungs, exchanging it for vital oxygen which is then delivered to the rest of the body.

This Inferior Vena Cava is a structure that demands respect and should be given a wide berth, if possible. Many surgeons reserve this attitude for the pancreas, but this large, thin-walled blood vessel can be most unforgiving.

For any readers unfamiliar with human anatomy, the body has several different types of vessels which carry blood and bodily fluids. Arteries are flexible, often muscular conduits which carry oxygenated blood under high pressure from the heart to body organs. The arteries progressively decrease in size as they branch into smaller arterioles and then capillaries, tiny thin-walled, porous vessels which only allow cells to pass in single file affording them the opportunity to deliver their wares (oxygen, nutrients, and such) to the body's organs, while picking up unwanted waste materials to be carried to the various outlets which will eliminate said waste. These capillaries then coalesce into veins which merge into larger and larger vessels, culminating in the Vena Cavas, of which there are two: Superior which carries blood from the head and arms to the heart, and Inferior which is the subject of this treatise. There is one other type of vessel, lymphatics, which carry fluid which has been dumped into the environment outside the usual circulatory system, eventually bringing it back into the network of arteries, veins, and capillaries.

This is not meant to be a dialogue on circulation, however. Rather, it is a discourse on the Inferior Vena Cava.

Getting back to my case, there it was, Big Blue, confronting me and my surgical skills. A lesser man would have been reduced to a tower of quivering Jell-o by the mere proximity of such a beast, but your humble correspondent is made of sterner stuff. It is true that one misstep, one single slip of the hand would lead to disaster, a hole in the suprahepatic Inferior Vena Cava.

Such an injury is very difficult to control and repair. This very short segment of the Inferior Vena Cava is right at the base of the heart. Bleeding from this area is akin to having a hole in the bottom of the heart. This is true because an injury to the suprahepatic Vena Cava really is a hole in the bottom of the heart. Every time the heart contracts its blood would be squeezed out this hole and the patient would bleed to death in short order. Traumatic injuries of this type are almost always fatal.

I did have to care for a patient with such an injury many years ago. Lydia had been in automobile accident. She arrived in our ER awake, alert, with a pulse, but we could not get a blood pressure. A peritoneal tap returned gross blood and she was whisked away to the OR. She was able to talk to us on the way and she had a weakly palpable femoral pulse.

As soon as we opened her abdomen we encountered blood, but where was it coming from? We packed all around the abdomen and then started our exploration. When I retracted downward on the liver, blood poured out, the hallmark of a retrohepatic or suprahepatic Vena Caval injury. The problem now was that our exploration had disrupted any tamponade (compression) that was limiting the bleeding from the injured vessel. Blood started to pour out with every contraction of her heart.

The treatment of such an injury requires placement of an atrio-caval shunt, a large tube which is passed through the right atrium of the heart into the Vena Cava and then secured so that the blood will flow through the tube and not the injured blood vessel, thus maintaining blood flow while allowing the surgical team to make repairs. Such a shunt can usually be placed in a few minutes. Lydia, however, did not have even a few minutes and she died of this lethal injury.

Excuse my digression, back to my encounter with Big Blue. The truth is that on every hiatal hernia repair, I am fully cognizant of the proximity of the Inferior Vena Cava. Often I see it clearly; sometimes I just wave at its presumed location. In this particular case, I took my usual care and placed each suture exactly where I wanted it, and was able to let sleeping monsters lie.

My first real encounter with Big Blue was many years ago, as a fourth-year surgical resident. I had been seeing a patient who had barely survived a complicated Gynecologic/Surgical operation. She was in the ICU and developed a pulmonary embolus, which is a blood clot from the legs or pelvis which breaks away and becomes lodged in the lungs, a life-threatening, sometimes fatal condition. She could not be placed on blood thinners because of the potential for bleeding which comes with these medications, therefore it was decided to place a "clip" on her Inferior Vena Cava. This clip allows blood to flow through the large vein, but prevents large, possibly fatal, clots from passing. This was before the use of intraluminal Vena Caval filters became the norm.

Normally, this procedure would be a Chief Resident case, but I managed to schedule it at a time when all the Chief residents would be tied up in a conference, thus affording me the opportunity to do this rarely performed surgical procedure. Up until that time, I had never done a similar operation and had never really worked on or around Big Blue. But, he who hesitates is lost. I read up on the technique and was filled with the bravado, confidence, and ignorance of youth. And, I pulled it off like a pro.

With two of my attending surgeons assisting, Big Blue was approached from the right side of the abdomen, the peritoneal structures were dissected off the retroperitoneum, and there I was, staring at the Inferior Vena Cava.

I gently began to spread and cut and spread until it was completely free. I slid the clip into place and closed it and that was it, my first successful encounter with Blue.

My Chief Resident, however, was really mad that I stole this case. Oh well, such are the fortunes of life.

There is another case that demonstrates just how dangerous and unforgiving the Inferior Vena Cava can be. It was actually one of my partners who started the surgery, which was the repair of a ruptured Abdominal Aortic Aneurysm. This is a condition where the major artery in the body has weakened and then burst, most often fatal with or without surgery.

I was called to see if I could lend a hand. I found him up to his elbows in blood, doing his best to stop the bleeding from the Vena Cava adjacent to the abdominal aorta. Multiple sutures had been placed and torn through, and now this giant vein was a macerated mess. With the patient already in extremis, all we could do was ligate, or tie off, the Vena Cava above its bifurcation and then go on and fix the aneurysm. Unfortunately, this patient didn't survive. Two lethal conditions simultaneously are too much for almost any individual or surgeon.

My fondest memory of battling the Vena Cava comes from Victor. Fond? Maybe not, but certainly challenging and interesting. He was forty-eight years old and came to see me because his abdomen was swelling. He was a mailman and he had noticed the prominence when his mailbag hit against his abdomen. He had never had any surgery or medical problems. He had only vague discomfort and no other symptoms. He was sent off for work up with an abdominal and pelvic CT Scan and basic blood tests.

The results of these tests revealed a large intrabdominal mass overlying his Inferior Vena Cava and right Renal Vein, while displacing the right colon and duodenum. He was mildly anemic, but otherwise his blood tests were normal. A needle biopsy was also done which revealed a spindle cell tumor. Sarcoma, a type of cancer, was suspected and surgery was scheduled.

Preoperative preparation included an arteriogram which provided a road map of the vessels supplying the tumor, a bowel prep because resection of a portion of the colon would likely be necessary along with all the routine antibiotics, type and cross match and such.

The big day (for the patient) arrived and he was whisked away to room five where he was epiduralized, catheterized, intubated, painted, and draped.

I made my usual grand entrance, with the theme from Rocky playing in the background, as my assistant, the circulating nurse, surgical tech, and anesthesiologist bowed, my freshly washed and sanitized hands held high.

In my dreams, maybe.

I was gowned and gloved and the surgery commenced.

A xiphoid to pubis midline incision brought us into the abdomen where the expected large mass was residing, pushing the colon up. The tumor was adherent to the mesentery of the right colon, but a bit of dissection revealed that the duodenum easily separated from the mass. With the duodenum out of the way and the tumor exposed, the operation could really begin. This mass was sitting on top of Big Blue.

I switched gears and began attacking this mass from behind the right kidney. The renal artery was not involved, but the mass was stuck to the right kidney, right Renal Vein, and the Inferior Vena Cava. Next, I started to gingerly dissect along Big Blue, starting on top of the right Iliac Vein which is the vein which joins with its partner on the left to form the Inferior Vena Cava. The tumor became adherent to Blue a few centimeters above this bifurcation.

Decision time was at hand. It was clear that a proper, curative resection would require removing a portion of Big Blue, as well as the right colon and right kidney. The big question loomed, however: Should the vena cava be ligated (closed completely by tying the divided ends) or reconstructed?

It wasn't really a difficult decision as I barely paused before asking to see what grafts were available. I chose an appropriately-sized "Platinum" graft and then really went to work. The terminal ileum was divided as was the transverse colon and the colonic mesentery (blood supply). Thus the colon was now free. The right kidney was dissected away from the surrounding tissue and the right renal artery ligated and divided. Finally the Vena Cava was dissected away from its resting place next to the aorta. Multiple lumbar veins were dissected free, clipped, and divided.

Finally I was left with only Big Blue. There was about seven centimeters of Vena Cava which would require removal. The big vein was clamped above its bifurcation and below the liver, divided and the cantaloupe-sized tumor was removed en bloc with the right colon, right kidney, and a portion of Big Blue.

Next it was time for reconstruction. Although I'm never thrilled about putting a prosthetic graft into a patient at the same time as a colon resection, there was little choice in Victor's case. His bowel was clean, however, and I made every attempt to limit the risk of contamination.

First, I rebuilt the Vena Cava. Some 5-0 Prolene suture, a bit of care, and the first anastomosis was done. A few minutes later and the second was completed. Now the moment of truth: the clamps were removed and, voila, blood was flowing through the graft and there was no leak. I put his colon back together next, doing my best to shield the new graft from any potential contamination.

Victor didn't turn a hair during his postoperative recovery. The tumor was found to be a liposarcoma, a type of cancer which probably originated in a single fat cell. After he had recovered from surgery and returned to work, I didn't give him much thought. As I tell many of my patients: "If you had surgery years ago and I remember you well, it means you either had a very unusual case or you had a significant complication. So be glad that I don't recall doing your gallbladder surgery fifteen years ago."

Victor did return, however, eight years after his surgery. He appeared to be in robust health but he had developed a hernia in his midline wound. I repaired this without any fuss, managing to stay well away from "Big Blue" during this particular operation.

NEVER TRUST A BONE DOCTOR

I suppose the title above is a bit facetious and I really don't mean it, but there have been times over the years when collaborating with my Orthopedic Surgery colleagues has caused sleepless nights. Some I didn't deserve.

Almost all these joint ventures have been on major trauma cases where severe bone injury has been paired with major vascular damage. Priority of repair, that is, who gets to go first, is a common discussion. The answer to the question depends on the patient and the injury. In general, life and limb threatening injuries take precedence over less serious traumas.

Such was the case of Mary, who suffered a closed fracture of her proximal tibia and fibula with associated occlusion of her popliteal artery and ischemia of her leg. The severe vascular injury could have led to Mary losing her leg and mending of the artery took precedence over the bony repair.

But, how could I have had the prescience to know that during the process of repairing the tibial fracture, the orthopedic surgeon would cause a bony fragment to compress the artery, which had just been patched and cleared of thrombus (a blood clot which was occluding the vessel)? The vessel became occluded again. My protests went unheeded and the bone doc said he couldn't do any better. I was forced to bite the bullet and redo the vascular repair utilizing a vein graft to bypass around the injured area.

At least I didn't have to drive back to the hospital. As a resident, experience taught me to never leave the vicinity until the bone doctor had driven his or her last screw, nailed the last nail, and placed the final skin staple. Only after checking my work would it be safe to leave, secure with the knowledge that my orthopedic colleague could not wreak anymore havoc.

Mary, by the way, recovered uneventfully.

Then there was Glenn.

It was a Friday night and I was not on call. My family and I had just walked in the door after dining out when my phone went off and there was a message. Dr. Black was consulting me to see Glenn, who was admitted to the hospital with a fracture of the proximal right humerus. The nurse was concerned because she could not feel a pulse and Glenn complained of his hand being numb. It was about eight o'clock in the evening.

I called and talked to the nurse and then headed in to the hospital. Glenn was in his mid fifties, lived with his parents, and had no significant medical problems other than being "a little slow" to use his expression. He told me he had tripped while on his parent's front porch and fallen down the three stairs to the sidewalk, landing on his right arm and shoulder. This had occurred at 11:00 a.m., now almost 10 hours earlier.

My exam confirmed that he had almost certainly injured his brachial artery. There was a large hematoma (collection of blood) in the upper arm and axilla, he could not move his hand, which was also numb, and there was no pulse in the arm, radial or brachial.

I called down to the OR, where they weren't very busy, and told the crew that Glenn needed surgery immediately. Next I called Dr. Black and reported my findings and he responded that he was on his way to the hospital.

I called the OR again and asked how quickly they would be ready, informing them, again, that this was a limb-threatening emergency and that the patient should have had his surgery hours before.

"We're opening now and anesthesia is on their way in," was the reply.

I have to admit I was a more than a little frustrated. Mostly it was the lack of attention that threatened to cause serious harm to Glenn that bothered me. It's not right for a patient to languish in the hospital with such an injury.

Dr. Black finally arrived.

"The ER physician told me it was an uncomplicated fracture. I had planned to fix it tomorrow," he explained without my ever asking a question or making a comment.

Finally, at 10:00, the OR team was ready and Glenn was wheeled down to surgery. The operation began about 30 minutes later. Glenn's arm had been ischemic for almost 12 hours.

I began to work, starting with an incision over the area where the subclavian artery emerges from beneath and behind the clavicle, following the rules and obtaining what's called "proximal control." What this means is that the artery is identified and dissected free in area closer to the heart than the injured area. Blood flows from the heart out to the organs under considerable pressure. Proximal control allows flow into the injured area to be interrupted should bleeding develop during the course of isolating the damaged artery.

I followed the artery out to the axilla, dissecting it free from the pectoralis major muscle and then into the upper arm where I encountered the large hematoma. This is where the artery had been bleeding before the pressure caused by the blood spilling into Glenn's tissues, along with the body's normal clotting mechanism, caused the hemorrhage to stop. If this mechanism had failed Glenn would have bled to death, but the human body is remarkable in its ability to fend off such calamity.

I evacuated the large blood clot and found one end of the transected artery, pulsing away, but not actively bleeding as the proximal artery had efficiently clotted.

Next I had to find the other end of the artery. Rather than start digging through the bloody, damaged tissue at the site of injury, I decided it would be more prudent to start at a site beyond the injury. The distal artery was easily dissected free and then followed back to the other injured end.

The two ends were a bit macerated and had retracted such that a direct end to end anastomosis (like reconnecting two ends of a pipe) was not feasible. Luckily I had the foresight to prep out Glenn's groin so that it was already sterile and I could harvest a segment of saphenous vein. This is the same vein commonly used for heart bypass surgery. Before starting on Glenn's leg I placed a shunt between the two divided ends of the injured artery, allowing blood to flow to the distal arm, thus giving the starved tissue a "drink" of blood, delivering oxygen and nutrients.

An adequate segment of vein was removed from his leg and the reconstruction proceeded without incident.

I added a fasciotomy to my procedure, which means I divided the fibrous tissue around the muscular compartments of the forearm to allow the muscle additional room to swell after it was reperfused, thus preventing what is termed "compartment syndrome." This condition can lead to muscle and nerve damage as the tissue swelling which can occur after prolonged periods of ischemia becomes confined by the tight, closed space of a muscular compartment.

I felt the strong pulse in the artery beyond my repair and saw that the muscle, although pale, looked viable and I believed Glenn would be left with a functional arm.

At this point I must add I had considered allowing Dr. Black to do his repair first. I could have placed the shunt to allow the arm to be perfused and then done the definitive repair after Dr. Black had finished. But, he assured me it was a simple fracture which was minimally displaced. He anticipated an uncomplicated ORIF (Open Reduction Internal Fixation). Being the trusting soul that I am, I performed the more vital arterial repair first.

However, I am not 100% naïve. I did stay around until Dr. Black finished. I'm glad I did. It was about 1:00 am when I lay down on the couch in the doctor's lounge and dozed off. Over the years, I've never slept well at the hospital, and I've always opted for driving home for a couple of hours' sleep in my own bed rather than getting an extra 30 minutes in the less comfortable confines of a hospital call room. In this case, however, it was fortunate that I did not leave.

The phone in the lounge rang at about 3:00 a.m.

"Dr. Gelber, you need to come check this arm," more of a command than request from the circulating nurse.

"Is Dr. Black finished?" I queried.

"Finished and gone, but you need to come."

"OK, OK, I'll be there in a minute."

I made a quick pit stop, donned my hat and mask and went back to the OR room where the surgical tech recounted the sad and tragic "saga of Glenn's repair."

"Well, he was doing the repair with a Rush Rod and it only took a few minutes. I thought we'd be home by 2:00, but then I picked up the arm and asked him if the Rod was supposed to come out the back of the arm? So he had to pull it out and that took a while. Then he had to do it again. I'm no Orthopedic Surgeon, but I don't think it's positioned very well. But, for what it's worth, he's done."

The circulator then spoke up.

"The hand looks white."

Sure enough there was no pulse or Doppler signal. So I was back at square one. I opened the wound and looked at my repair. There was an excellent pulse at the site of the repair and for at least three or four centimeters distal. I started dissecting farther and it wasn't long before I found the problem.

Dr. Black had not only driven that Rod through the back of Glenn's arm, but he had also managed to put it through the brachial artery at a point beyond the original injury. So, I repaired the artery a second time. At least I didn't have to do another fasciotomy.

I finished at around 5:00 a.m. Glenn woke and had much improved function of his hand. He could move it and there was some sensation. He maintained good perfusion of his arm, but did have to have the orthopedic reconstruction revised at a later date. Eventually he regained 100% full, normal function of his arm and hand.

Dr. Black never talked about this particular case with me. A couple of years later, he gave up the practice of Orthopedics. He was, overall, a competent surgeon and his retirement from Orthopedics was for personal and health reasons, unrelated to Glenn's case.

I hope that anyone who reads these words does not believe that I have no regard or respect for my Orthopedic colleagues. I could never do what they do and most are excellent physicians and surgeons. They do, however, have a singlemindedness in their approach to their patients. Their job is to fix, reconstruct, and otherwise mend broken, worn out, and degenerated bones and joints. Orthopedic surgical procedures are designed to stay away from vital structures such as nerves, major blood vessels, and other organs which are soft and not amenable to nails, screws, and plates.

What I've learned is that injuries and medical conditions which bring me into the Orthopedic Surgeon's realm require that I maintain my utmost vigilance. And, never completely trust a bone doctor.

UGI BLEEDING

During residency, one of my attending surgeons stated that he hated the phrase "GI Bleeding."

"It's gastrointestinal hemorrhage," he would preach.

The assembled congregation of residents would nod their heads in unison as if Dr. O had just predicted the exact date of the second coming. Like most religious experiences, this dogma lasted until we left the conference room. Later in the day, the Chief resident would ask me to go see the GI bleeder in ICU.

GI bleeding is a very common problem. Vomiting blood, bloody diarrhea, dark blood, bright red blood, coffee ground blood, occult blood are all manifestations of blood loss from the gastrointestinal tract. The source can be anywhere from mouth to anus. The cause ranges from ulcer to tumor to infection to vascular malformations along with many other conditions.

Most of the time the bleeding stops or can be controlled without major surgery. Often this bleeding is intermittent, affording the treating physicians the luxury of time to track down the exact site and cause. Armed with such information the proper therapy can be initiated, be it medication, endoscopy, or surgery.

Sometimes, however, this bleeding is profuse and immediately life threatening. Annette was one such case.

Annette was a physician, a psychiatrist to be exact. Still, being a psychiatrist did not make her immune to human frailties. Her weakness was alcohol. Specifically, she drank almost a quart of vodka daily. I was called by Dr. S., the GI consultant, as he was about to do an endoscopy, an esophagogastroduodenoscopy, or EGD.

"She's been hypotensive," he reported, "and is passing bright red blood from her rectum and NG tube. We've already transfused six units of packed cells and her hemoglobin is staying at eight."

"I'm on my way in." I answered.

Why do these disasters always happen at night?

It was 10:00 p.m.

I arrived with the endoscopy in progress. On my way I had called the OR and, luckily, the crew was already there, just finishing another case. I advised them to stick around. I had a feeling about Annette, a feeling which whispered she would be going to the OR sooner rather than later.

"There's a lot of blood," Dr. S. reported. "I can't see exactly where it's coming from."

"You're right, there is a lot of blood." I could see nothing but blood and clots filling up Annette's stomach. "I think she's going to need surgery. Any guesses as to the exact source?"

"Duodenum, probably an ulcer in the bulb," Dr. S. concluded.

"OK, I'll start there."

With the EGD finished I finally was able to get a good look at Annette. What was striking about her appearance was her color, rather, her lack of color. She was white. Not in the Caucasian sense, no, she was white in a ghostly way, as if she had suffered a prolonged encounter with a vampire. Her blood pressure was 70/0 and her heart was zipping along at 140.

"Pump the blood in," I ordered.

I called the OR to officially schedule her surgery, then talked with Annette's husband. 30 minutes later, she was on the OR table.

We continued to pour packed RBC's along with other blood products into Annette as she was put to sleep and the surgery started.

Need to work quickly and get this bleeding stopped.

I entered her abdomen as rapidly as possible through a generous upper midline incision. There was a bit of watery fluid in the abdomen and everything looked as pale as her skin.

Dracula would starve here.

Her blood pressure dropped to 50 as I opened her stomach, carrying the gastrostomy through the pylorus and extending it to include the first part of the duodenum. The stomach was full of dark clotted blood, which was evacuated, filling up a large basin. Bright red blood was welling up from just beyond the pylorus.

There's the culprit.

A large ulcer filled the first part of the duodenum and blood was pumping out from its base.

"2-0 silk, please," I requested.

The surgical tech slapped the needle driver and suture in my hand. First one stitch, then another, and another, and the bleeding stopped.

"Probably the gastroduodenal artery," I announced to no one in particular. "A couple of more stitches, a vagotomy, close this big hole in the stomach, and then we will be done."

I over-sewed the ulcer from inside the duodenum, watched it for a minute to be sure there was no bleeding and then began to close the long gastrostomy.

It's going to be quite a long pyloroplasty. What is the name? Finney, I think?

A pyloroplasty means that the pylorus, which is the muscle at the end of the stomach which controls how quickly or slowly food is released into the small intestine, is reshaped, altered, or divided. Most commonly the procedure involves a short longitudinal incision carried from the stomach, through the pylorus, and onto the first part of the duodenum. This is then closed transversely, thus dividing the pylorus and enlarging the opening at the end of the stomach. This is the common Heineke-Mickulicz pyloroplasty. If a longer opening is made in the stomach and duodedum and closed transversely, that is called a Finney. Another type is the Jaboulay.

Annette's pyloroplasty came together without any fuss. Her blood pressure was up to 100/50. I reinforced the pyloroplasty suture line with my old friend, the omentum. Next, I approached the gastrointestinal junction, looking for the vagus nerves. The left lobe of the liver was mobilized and retracted, the peritoneum over the junction of the esophagus and stomach was opened, and I began to search for the vagus nerves.

Using my fingers to bluntly dissect, I felt the nasogastric tube in her esophagus, then gradually worked my fingers around. The stomach was placed on some traction, pulling it downwards. Around the backside of the esophagus, I felt a tight wire-like structure. Continuing to use finger dissection, this structure was freed from the tissue surrounding it and brought out from its hiding place, and grasped with a clamp. It was then clip, clip, cut, and the posterior vagotomy was done. Next, I looked for another wire running along the front of the esophagus. Once again, downward traction on the stomach, a bit of dissection with fingers, and a clamp, and the anterior vagus nerve was isolated, clipped, and a portion excised.

Annette's blood pressure was 110; heart rate was down to 98. I closed her up and she was wheeled back to the ICU.

Another life prolonged. That's four this week.

As she was being tucked away in the ICU, I went to talk to her family: husband, three children, a sister, and niece.

"Well, the surgery is all done," I began. "She had quite a big ulcer which was pouring out blood. But we fixed that and she's back in the ICU. Her blood pressure is normal and her heart rate is down. We'll have to wait and see if any new problems develop."

"Is she going to live?" the sister asked.

"I hope so. She's still not out of the woods. The bleeding is stopped, but she could develop problems with other organs. Her kidneys or lungs may have been affected. There could be some effects on her brain. Or, she could just wake up with no other issues and be out of here in four or five days."

The surgery finished at around midnight. I stayed around while she woke up to be sure she was stable. I gave her two more units of blood, talked with the Pulmonary specialist and her attending physician.

Annette remained stable. Her blood pressure came up to 130/80, heart rate dropped to 90, she was making some urine, and her oxygen saturation was 100%. Finally, she was opening her eyes and able to follow commands. I left for home around 1:30 a.m.

Annette didn't bleed anymore. The following morning her NG tube had the much hoped for yellow-green drainage of bile. She became less dependent on the ventilator and was extubated later that day. Her BUN and Creatinine did rise, reaching 40 and 2.5 before returning to normal.

Looks like she'll recover without any major sequelae.

It wasn't to be all smooth sailing, however.

Why are such things called complications?

"She doesn't seem to be all there, mentally," her husband reported.

"Probably the alcohol, rather the withdrawal of alcohol," I surmised.

Annette was seeing things, picking at unseen bugs in the air.

"Look at that rat!!" she screamed, causing her nurse to come running.

"Get them off of me!!!" she yelled even louder, cowering under her blanket.

The battle against the demons brought out by her unsettled mind went on for about five days.

"She's suffering from a number of shocks to her body," I tried to reassure her husband. "She almost bled to death, she was a heavy drinker, she's received a lot of other medication. I think she'll get back to normal, but it may take some time."

Her husband nodded his head and then added, "You know, even before all this happened, she had moments when she didn't seem quite all there. There were times when I would catch her sitting alone talking to no one. She always laughed and said it was just a joke and I dismissed it."

Maybe she needed to see a Psychiatrist.

As if he could read my thoughts, her husband added, "She did see a Psychiatrist. She was supposed to be on some sort of psych meds, but I think she drank instead of taking any medication. Alcohol was her drug of choice. Tell me, Dr. G, do you really think she'll ever be back to her old self?"

"I wish I knew for sure. I can tell you that my patients in the past who have been sick like Annette and recover, usually get back to their old selves. They feel like they have lost part of their life to being ill, like it's a big void, but everyone has recovered," I replied.

Annette was seen by a psychiatric consultant. She was started on medication, but continued to be confused. She was transferred to another facility after about 2 weeks, stable in every way except mentally.

"Bring Annette to my office in about two weeks," I instructed. "I'll need to see how she's doing from the surgery."

"Thanks for all you did for her, Dr. G, saving her life and all." Her husband shook my hand and left.

It was almost six weeks later when Annette showed up in my office.

She came with her husband.

"They tell me I should thank you for saving my life," she said as she shook my hand.

"You were very sick when I was called," I answered. "How are you feeling now?"

"I still get tired a lot. I haven't been able to work."

"Eating OK, no fever, bowels OK?"

"Yes, yes, all that is just fine. Sometimes I feel like I'm in fog, though. I'll be thinking about something and then, nothing, my mind just goes blank. It's like something has taken an eraser and wiped out everything in my head. It takes a minute and then the thoughts come back."

"Give it some time and you'll probably get back to normal," I predicted.

Annette and her husband left. It was the last time I saw either one.

Give it some time.

These are words I've used over and over. Doctors can intervene in an illness with medication or surgery, do what we think is best to arrest the disease process, repair the damage done by cancer or injury, but the body still has to heal. Organs need time to recover, to rebuild, to return to their normal state.

Time.

It is the doctor's greatest ally.

CHRISTMAS EVE

It was Christmas and I was on call. Christmas Eve was on Thursday, the office was closed and my partners had left town, including Dr. W. who should have been on back up call. He begged me to cover solo as his daughter had just given birth to his first grandchild and he desperately wanted to spend Christmas with her family.

"Go on, I'll be OK," I told him.

Even Laura and the kids were gone, spending the holiday with her family in Dallas.

It was just me and the dogs and the birds.

And the Emergency Room.

I was on call for the ER Christmas Eve, but not Christmas Day.

Even if it's busy Christmas Eve, I should get some rest the next day.

Two things I didn't plan.

The ER decided that that Christmas Eve would be the busiest night of surgical diseases it had seen in the five years I'd been in practice.

And, a stomach bug.

It started at 1:00 p.m.

"I've got a twenty-year-old male, I'm pretty sure has appendicitis," Dr. M. reported.

"Ok, the OR crew is here and not very busy, I'll be over to see him shortly," I answered.

Something's not right.

I stood up and felt light headed for a moment and then a headache began to brew above my eyes. I sat down for a minute.

Maybe I just need something to drink.

I fished a Coke out of the doctor's lounge fridge and then made my way to the ER, feeling a little better.

Manuel was twenty, healthy and had classic appendicitis. This was in the days before routine CT scanning for suspected appendicitis. The OR crew whisked him over to surgery and an hour later he was safely tucked away in the Recovery room, while his nasty, inflamed appendix floated in a jar of formalin.

Maybe it's something I ate.

My head was pounding now and I was sure I had a fever. A wave of nausea started at my feet, rose to my head and finally settled in my abdomen. My stomach began to cramp.

Then my beeper went off: Call 1440. The ER.

"Got a guy down here with a big perirectal abscess," this time Dr. H was calling.

Mike was 60 and had an abscess the size of an apple adjacent to his anus.

"It started the size of a pea a few days ago. I thought it would go away, but it just got bigger and bigger and hurt more and more."

That's all I need right now. I think the sweet aroma will kill me.

The OR crew picked him and I spent Mike's twenty-minute operation breathing through my mouth, hoping that I would not vomit until the end of the case.

I should call someone to take over. I'm sure my temperature is a hundred and three.

Mike was safely packed away in the Recovery Room as I called one of my partners.

"Sorry, I'm up in Austin. Maybe Dr. E is around."

Dr. E. was in Europe. Dr. S. was in San Antonio.

You did agree to work these two days without backup. Everything will be fine. It's only ER call for one night. Maybe one of the guys outside our group will take pity on me.

"It's Christmas Eve."

"No."

"NO."

"Hell No."

Not much spirit of giving among them. I took three Advil. My beeper went off as soon as they hit my stomach.

"1440."

It's going to be a long night.

"Seventy-year-old female with abdominal pain, nausea, and vomiting for three days. WBC is 22,000 and she's got forty bands. Heartrate is one twenty. X-ray shows multiple air fluid levels and dilated small bowel. Only previous surgery was hysterectomy twenty years ago."

Just great, another surgery. Maybe that Advil will kick in soon.

I made the short walk down the hall to the ER and found Alison. She was just as presented. She had a tender abdomen along with the other signs which suggested she had ischemic bowel.

"Looks like you need surgery," I explained.

"But, my daughter is coming to visit, from Australia," she explained. "I haven't seen her in five years."

"Well, she'll have to come a little farther to see you. I think part of your intestine is dying. If we don't do surgery you may not ever see her again," I explained. "OK," she gave in meekly. "I know you're right. This pain has only been getting worse." We had Alison up in surgery about thirty minutes later. At least the Advil was kicking in. I felt better. I was a little sweaty which made me think the fever was breaking and my headache was gone.

I opened Alison up through her previous lower midline wound and found a loop of small bowel trapped between the abdominal wall and a single thick adhesion. About twenty centimeters of bowel was being strangled. One little snip and it was free. The dark hemorrhagic bowel began to turn red and then pink. I wrapped warm towels around it and left it alone for five minutes, then five more minutes. After these ten minutes it looked much happier, pinker, with a few dark blotches which were fading away. A few minutes later I was sure it would all survive. I tucked it back in her abdomen and closed her up.

My beeper went off again.

"2700."

At least it's not the ER.

It was ICU.

"I'm calling about Mr. J. Dr. E. did a colon resection 10 days ago. He just coughed and now there's bowel hanging out from his wound."

Here we go again.

Why is Mr. J. still in the ICU 10 days after surgery? I wondered out loud.

His nurse must have heard me.

"He had an MI two days ago and has been having all sorts of arrhythmias. SVT, PVC's, PAC's, A. Fib.," she recited.

"Regular alphabet soup, it seems," I answered. "What's he doing now?"

He's been in sinus for the last couple of hours. Dr. M. is his cardiologist. He was here a few minutes ago."

I called Dr. M. and explained the situation.

"Do what you need to do. I'll be around to take care of his heart."

The OR team came to get him about twenty minutes later.

Mr. J. was 78 years old. He had been recovering uneventfully from his right colon resection when he developed chest pain and suffered the Myocardial Infarction. Cardiac cath had been done which revealed diffuse disease not amenable to stenting or surgery. There were some notes in the chart about a pacemaker, but no decision had been made.

"We need to bring you down to surgery and put you back together," I explained.

"Why did this happen?" he asked me.

"I can't say for sure. When we have you asleep I'll be able to see why. Maybe a stitch broke or maybe there's some infection which weakened the tissue. Whatever the cause, we can't leave you with your guts hanging out."

"Should be pretty quick," I told Anesthesia.

He just shook his head. He placed an arterial line before putting Mr. J. to sleep.

At surgery it looked like the running suture my partner had used had broken. The fascia all looked strong with no sign of infection. I felt a little guilt because I had convinced my partner that the single layer closure with a running stitch was the best way to put an abdomen back together. The evidence supported me, but if the suture breaks, such closing technique is definitely not the best.

I took a quick look around the abdomen before closing the belly. All looked to be in order.

"I need a bunch of #2 Mersilene and some rubber bolsters and a #1 PDS," I requested.

I placed each Mersilene retention suture about three centimeters apart, try to put them so that each suture would be outside the peritoneum. Retention sutures are large, heavy stitches which go through all layers of the abdominal wall. They will keep an abdomen together even under the worst circumstances; at least that is what surgeons hope. I also closed him with another running suture to just his fascia.

Belt and suspenders.

Mr. J. didn't turn a hair during his 35-minute operation. He was brought back to the ICU, appearing none the worse for having to go through a second operation.

"No one ever suffered from a celiotomy," one of my attending surgeons during residency once said. I was never sure I believed this after seeing patients return with hernias, suffer aspiration pneumonia secondary to post op ileus or require re-exploration because of bleeding from an artery in the abdominal wall.

Any operation carries risks and benefits and these must be weighed when any surgery is considered. That is one of my rules. I know I am not an academic type, but I do have almost 30 year's experience.

Mr. J was stable. I wasn't sure I could say the same for myself. My joints ached, my head was about to explode, and I felt like there was a 20-pound weight sitting in my stomach.

Advil had worked for a short while. Maybe some Tylenol will help. And, a few moments repose.

I lay down in the call room and almost fell asleep.

Beep, beep.

1440.

"We've got an 86-year-old man with a cold leg. Started suddenly about four hours ago," Dr. H. reported. "He's in atrial fibrillation which is new. EKG from two months ago was sinus. There are no pulses or Doppler signal below the femoral on the right."

"I'll be over," I groaned.

It was almost 8:00 p.m.

Gerald's leg was white.

"Never had any problem before, Doc. Just got cold and really hurt about 4:00. Don't feel much now," he said.

Gerald had no circulation below the femoral artery. The proximal thigh was warm, but the rest of the leg was cold, white, lifeless.

He almost certainly had an arterial embolus, which is a blood clot which probably formed in his heart, broke loose, and lodged in his right femoral artery. I saw no need for further studies.

New onset atrial fibrillation in previously asymptomatic patient who now had severe ischemia spelled arterial embolus. This is in contrast to thrombosis. An embolus is a clot which moves from one part of the body to another; in this case heart to femoral artery. Thrombosis occurs in arteries which already have narrowing secondary atherosclerosis. The narrowed artery gradually builds up a clot until it completely occludes or becomes thrombosed. Often, acute thrombosis has less severe symptoms because the gradual narrowing allows collateral vessels to develop, a situation I describe as "the highway being closed, but the side streets are open."

Acute thromboses, at least in the peripheral circulation, usually allow time to properly evaluate the patient with imaging studies, without compromising the viability of the affected limb. An embolus to the leg, like Gerald's, does not afford time for collateral circulation to develop and is a limb-threatening condition which is best treated with emergency embolectomy, which is opening up the artery and removing the offending clot. At least that's how it was done back in the old pre-endo-vascular intervention days.

At least the Tylenol is kicking in.

The hammer which had been beating the inside of my skull had receded to a vague ache in the back of my head. I was able to sit upright without my stomach spilling out into my lap as the OR crew fetched Gerald. The Tylenol's effect peaked as I made my appearance in the OR while Gerald was being prepped.

The surgery was as straightforward as could be. Gerald was pretty thin, I was down to the artery as soon as I made the skin incision. There was a pulse in the artery until it divided into the superficial and deep femoral branches. I made short order of dissecting the artery free.

Clamp, clamp, clamp, cut, and there was the "bullet" or embolus lodged at the division of the common femoral artery. I fished it out, passed the balloon-tipped Fogarty catheter up and down the artery, fishing out a few small clots, and then closed him up.

Gerald's circulation was restored, marked by palpable pulses in the posterior tibial and dorsalis pedis arteries in the right foot, which was now pink and gradually warming up.

Another leg saved. Time to go home and get some sleep.

Beep… Beep.

1440. I think I hate that number.

"We've got an MVA, heart rate is 140 and BP is 90. Fractured ribs on the left. CT shows a ruptured spleen and a lot of blood in the belly. Also a 20-year-old male with Right Lower Quadrant abdominal pain for three days and WBC of 21,000."

So much for sleep. Three more Advil, perhaps?

Mona had driven her car into a pole. She had been drinking and there was something about a fight with her boyfriend. Despite fluid and blood resuscitation, she remained hypotensive and surgery was indicated.

Guadalupe was another classic case of appendicitis. He would have to wait until I finished with Mona.

I battled a wave of nausea after taking the Advil, which passed. The subjective sense of fever which had returned also abated as the medication began to take effect.

Mona was wheeled into surgery and I started with a generous midline incision. The blood was evacuated, and the left upper quadrant was packed with lap pads as I explored the rest of the abdomen.

Liver, bowel, stomach, retroperitoneum, all clean.

Let's take care this spleen and get out of here.

I reached my hand back behind the spleen and pulled it down. The laceration was in the mid-portion and extended into the hilum. I manually compressed the area of bleeding as I divided the attachments to the diaphragm and freed the splenic flexure of the colon.

Then it was clamp, clamp, cut, clamp, clamp, cut, clamp, clamp, cut, until I threw the spleen into the waiting basin.

"2-0 silk on a needle, please, a bunch of them," I requested.

Each vessel was stitched, and the splenic artery and vein were each sutured twice. I checked to be sure I hadn't inadvertently lopped off the tail of the pancreas, then checked for bleeding, washed everything out, checked the bowel again, and then closed her up.

It was midnight when she was settled in the ICU. I went to lie down until Guadalupe was ready for his appendectomy.

I hope this is it. Everything aches.

It was the last emergency for the night, but it also was not my usual 20-minute appendectomy.

Guadalupe presented me with a twisted mass of omentum, small bowel, and pus surrounding his three-day-old, ruptured, gangrenous appendix. I spent two and a half hours teasing and cajoling the inflamed mass of tissue away from the foul appendix. The inflammation on the appendix extended all the way to the cecum which required me to mobilize the right colon enough to find an area where there was no inflammation. I was able to staple across this area and remove the appendix in three separate pieces, doing my best to insure that the entire organ was excised. Guadalupe's abdomen was washed with a large volume of saline and then closed.

It was 3:00 a.m. when I finally said "Thank you" to the unseen transcriptionist on the other end of the phone line for the last time.

I need to lie down and get some rest.

I looked up and saw a decrepit man staring back at me from the mirror, eyes puffy and bloodshot, cheeks flushed, hair a tousled jumble. I took two more Tylenol and lay down in the call room for about 20 minutes. I started to feel better and decided I'd rather sleep in my own bed. The ER assured me there was nothing brewing.

I was in my bed by 4:00 and slept for about four hours before I decided it was time to face the new day.

I suppose one could say that I survived this night on call. Before I passed into a state of oblivion, I thought about the day. Seven true emergencies were treated, not counting myself. The amazing thing is that I never felt ill while operating. Each surgery was carried out in an orderly and expeditious manner. Advil, Tylenol, and endogenous epinephrine kept my concentration and dexterity at their usual high levels and I can't say that any of these patients received substandard care.

Seven emergencies. Seven operations. Seven excellent outcomes.

Was it the medication? Perhaps. My own fantastic surgical skill? Doubtful. Divine Intervention? Possibly.

The way it all turned out, maybe I should be sick more often.

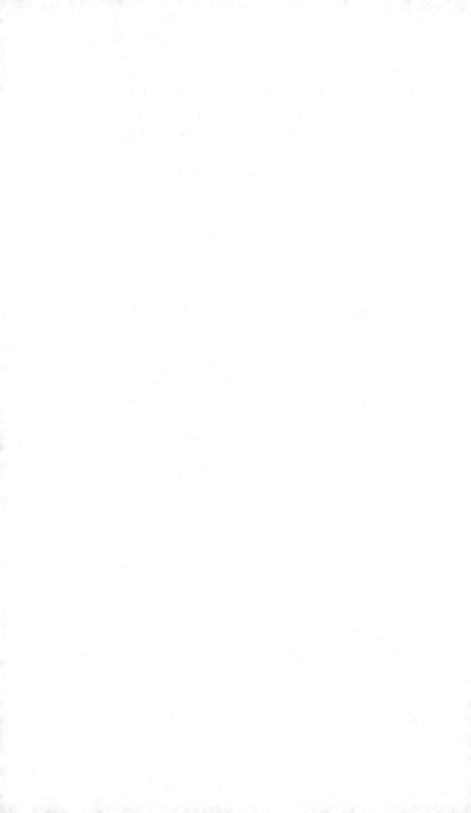

A SENSE OF WHERE YOU ARE

Years ago I read a book about former US Senator and basketball great, Bill Bradley, which was titled, "A Sense of Where You Are."

The title derived from a basketball move he could perform which had him drive along the baseline to blindly shoot a reverse layup. He described how he had developed a sort of sixth sense which allowed him to make this shot, even though he couldn't see the basket. He had played so much basketball and knew the court so well that he had developed "a sense of where you are."

This saying burrowed out of the back of my brain into my consciousness the other day as I was doing a parathyroidectomy. Now don't get the idea that I perform surgery blindly. But, parathyroid surgery sometimes requires a sixth sense to track down these pesky little glands. For those of you unfamiliar with the anatomy of the human neck, the parathyroids are four separate glands which hide behind the thyroid gland. A normal parathyroid is about 4-5 millimeters in diameter. Each gland is described relative to its position to the thyroid gland, which is a butterfly shaped organ sitting in the middle of the neck. Thus, there are right and left, upper and lower parathyroid glands, depending on their position behind or adjacent to the thyroid gland. Sometimes, (often) these parathyroids like to hide. They may be lower in the neck, closer to the carotid artery or even lower, in the mediastinum (behind the breast bone). It's sort of like they know someone is searching for them, they don't want to be found and they decide to take shelter away from their usual residence.

I've done a lot of parathyroid surgeries over the years. Most of the time preoperative testing provides some guidance as to where the abnormal gland is residing. But, these preop scans usually only tell me right or left, upper or lower. I still have to find the offending little beast. This is where it is helpful to have a good sense of where one is.

So, I start by getting the thyroid out of the way which requires dividing a few veins which are collectively called the middle thyroid vein. Then it's time to look, first for "the nerve," the recurrent laryngeal nerve which causes our vocal cords to move, but also for bulges rising from beneath fat which don't look like they belong or send me a signal which says, "there's something hiding under here." The vast majority of the time it is this "something looks out of place" sense that leads me straight to the offending parathyroid gland. After that, it is relatively simple to remove the gland and have my friendly neighborhood Pathologist confirm it is abnormal.

Unfortunately, it's not always easy.

Vince was in his sixties when he came to me with long-standing hypercalcemia and very elevated parathyroid hormone levels, lab tests which led to the diagnosis of primary hyperparathyroidism. Surgery was recommended. His preoperative imaging studies were all normal.

Despite this, he still needed surgery, only with him I had nothing to tell me where to look. So I started first in the left lower position, which is the easiest area to explore. I was heartened as I saw a nodule that appeared to be separate from the thyroid gland. However, as my dissection continued, it became clear that this nodule was part of the thyroid itself. Onward went the dissection. In the left upper thyroid I found a tiny, normal appearing parathyroid, about 2 mm in diameter. I looked at the right side and saw a tiny gland behind the lower pole of the thyroid. I didn't find anything that looked like parathyroid on the upper end. I did identify the recurrent laryngeal nerves and both carotid arteries on both sides. I went back to searching. Perhaps behind the mound of fat next to the right carotid. There was something there. As I removed it my heart sank. It looked more like a lymph node. I sent it off anyway and was not surprised when the Pathologist confirmed that it was a lymph node and not parathyroid.

Where are you, you irritating, mischievous sprite?

Well, maybe down in the mediastinum, which is behind the sternum. So I start pulling tissue, mostly fat, out of the upper chest. Nothing, nothing and more nothing. I had been searching for more than two hours without success.

Maybe it's time to give up, do more tests, perhaps?

I looked a bit more, farther down in the chest, more towards the middle. I found something. It looked like a parathyroid, kidney bean size, shape, and color. Out it came and off it went to the lab.

"Hyperplastic parathyroid."

Thank you, Pathologist.

Vince's parathyroid hormone was checked before we woke him up. It fell from a preop level of 2200 down to 500 and then to 40 prior to discharge. His calcium levels dropped to normal. He was cured.

This "sense of where you are" is important in surgeries beside parathyroidectomy. Every operation requires knowledge of anatomy, with all its variants. Plus, surgeons need to be aware of distortions of normal anatomy due to cancer or inflammation or trauma.

Operations require dissection and cutting and more dissection, all the time knowing that important structures may be lurking nearby. Colon surgery requires the surgeon to be aware that the ureter and iliac artery and vein are just behind the bowel; biliary tract surgery requires cognizance of the proximity of the common bile duct, hepatic artery, inferior vena cava, portal vein, duodenum and pancreas. The spleen is always hanging around gastric and pancreatic surgery. A sense of where you are becomes important in almost all operations.

All surgeons must be aware of the potential pitfalls of each operation they perform. Some surgeons have this "sixth sense" that tells them when to be extra careful, to dissect gingerly, as catastrophe and disaster may be only a small snip away.

This "sense of where you are" is honed by experience. It isn't "evidence based" but it is real and helps make surgery cleaner, quicker, and safer.

UR (AMAZING) ANUS

I know it's supposed to be one of the forbidden parts, an area hidden and unmentionable, but, I have to say it, the anus is a remarkable organ. Think about it. It is so sensitive and functions with remarkable competence.

The human alimentary tract starts at the mouth. This beginning is also super sensitive. Lips are designed to take on so many shapes and attitudes, perfect for sipping, pouting, smiling and, most important, kissing. The tongue is also super sensitive. A tiny hair floating on the tongue is so annoying, you just have to reach in inside your mouth and retrieve it.

But it is the exit from the alimentary tract which is amazing. We treat it in such a derogatory manner, hiding it and putting it to use in the most private way, giving it profane names like a—hole or butthole, but the anus is far more than a mere opening.

Anatomically the anus consists of the anoderm, underlying sphincter muscles, blood vessels, nerves, and so much more. It only opens when necessary. And, if something isn't right, it lets the owner know. A tiny amount of mucus or stool left behind persistently irritates until it is cleansed away. The anus exists in a state bombarded by bacteria, yet fights off infection with aplomb. And, if wayward bacteria manages to set up shop and an infection is established, it is usually kept localized, rather than invading the entire body.

And, it is discerning. It distinguishes between gas and substance, sometimes releasing one, while holding the other, until the proper moment.

One must agree that the anus works wonders and is vastly superior to any alternative. But, when it betrays us we know it. Hemorrhoids, fissures, abscesses can be excruciatingly painful or cause profuse bleeding. We know when something is wrong and it is time to see the Proctologist.

Which brings me to Penny.

Penny came to the office one day, brought by her husband, with the complaint of "Anal Condyloma." At least that's what my schedule said. Anal Condyloma, which are warts caused by the human papilloma virus, are not uncommon. Most of the time there are a few warts, sometimes up to twenty of thirty. The vast majority of cases are sexually transmitted.

There is no question that Penny had anal condyloma. There were not just a few. Collectively they were the size of a large cauliflower.

"How long have you had this problem," I wondered.

"About a year. I kept thinking it would get better and go away," she answered. "I can't sit, I'm in such pain. Can't you do something?"

When I examined her I saw wart after wart on top of wart. The entire jumble was very clean, however, a testament to the doting care of her dedicated husband.

I'm not sure what to do with this? And it may be a cancer.

I had never seen such an extensive mass of anal condyloma. I measured the diameter at 24 centimeters.

Maybe treat it like a squamous cell carcinoma. Begin with radiation and or chemotherapy. Shrink it down to a manageable size.

I called Dr. H, one of my Oncology consultants, and described the situation.

After much discussion, we decided that a biopsy was in order.

Penny was in such pain and so tender that any sort of biopsy without general anesthesia was unthinkable. I scheduled her for exam under anesthesia with biopsy for later in the week, gave her some pain medication and told her and her husband I'd see them in a couple of days.

"Don't worry. We will do everything we can to fix this problem," I reassured them.

But I wasn't so sure.

Two days later, Penny was being wheeled into the OR for what was to be a short procedure. She went to sleep and then it was time to position her for the biopsy. She was put in lithotomy position, which meant her legs were elevated and separated in "candy cane" stirrups. There was a distinct widening of the eyes of the OR personnel when they first glimpsed the huge flowering mass enveloping her anus.

"I've never seen anything like that."

"How could she let it go so far?"

"Is it cancer?"

I politely answered their questions and then proceeded to the task.

I gave Penny a thorough exam while she was asleep. The large mass was confined to the skin. As expected, there was no extension into the rectum. Condyloma only grow in squamous mucosa, therefore there should not be any rectal involvement. However, if the condyloma had morphed into a cancer, then it could grow and spread anywhere.

After the exam, I excised a portion of the mass from two separate areas, one at the periphery, removing some normal skin with the mass, and the second from the interior of the mass. The entire procedure lasted about ten minutes.

The biopsy revealed condyloma acuminata with dysplasia, and focal well differentiated squamous cell carcinoma.

Penny began treatment with chemo/radiation ten days later. I did not see her for three months. A call came from Dr.H, her Oncologist.

"Well, we've done as much as we can with Penny. She's had some response. Her recent CT reveals some enlarged lymph nodes in her groins. She's as ready as she will ever be for surgery."

Penny came to the office a few days later. Her response to therapy was not what I'd hoped for. The tumor mass had shrunk, but only by about a third. Instead of a large cauliflower, it was a medium cantaloupe.

"There is some improvement," I explained. "How do you feel?"

"About the same," she answered, as her husband nodded in agreement.

"It looks like it's time for surgery," I added. "The operation is what is called an abdominoperineal resection. This means removal of the rectum and anus. You will have a permanent colostomy. That means you'll have a bag instead of going to the bathroom in the usual manner."

"As long as I can sit," she said.

"You should feel better," I added.

I hope she heals OK. At least this preop treatment did some good. It looks like I should be able to close her bottom.

A week later Penny was back in the OR, asleep, once again in lithotomy position, only this time there was no oohing and aahing from the OR staff. It was a big surgery and everyone was on their toes.

The surgery began with a midline incision and the initial exploration of her abdomen. As expected, nothing unusual was found. Specifically, there was no sign of tumor. The abdominal portion of this APR was as straightforward as could be expected.

The abdominoperineal resection is an operation which removes the rectum and anus, almost exclusively performed for malignancy, most commonly adenocarcinoma of the rectum. Other indications would be cancer of the anus, which was Penny's condition, and any other cancer which involved the distal rectum or anus. The surgery is performed through an abdominal incision and a perineal incision; the perineum is the area which includes the anus and external genitals.

One could ask: Why not remove just Penny's tumor with the anus? After all, her cancer did not involve the rectum. Unfortunately, such an operation would leave Penny with a miserable existence. The anus gives us control. Its sphincter muscles allow us to decide when and where we defecate. Now imagine life without an anus, one where the rectum is connected to the perineal skin. It would be like having a colostomy in that area, except there would be no bag. There would be uncontrolled passage of stool, anytime, without warning. And trying to put a colostomy bag in that area would be impossible. Removal of the anus, means a permanent colostomy. It is, however, possible to remove the rectum,

210 | Amazing Days, Endless Nights

leave the anus, and avoid a permanent colostomy. Such "ileoanal" procedures are most commonly done for severe inflammatory bowel disease. A complete description of such procedures is for textbooks and is not part of Penny's story. The abdominal portion of Penny's surgery proceeded without a hitch. The rectum was divided where it joined the sigmoid colon and it was dissected free as distally as I could manage through the abdomen. I've learned, over the years, that the more dissection which can be done through the abdomen the less frustration I will suffer when I execute the perineal portion. I managed to dissect down to the levator muscles via the abdomen, which is almost to the anus. Even so, I knew that the challenge was yet to come: removing that mass of tumor and warts.

Having finished the abdominal portion of the dissection I sat down between Penny's legs and stared at the tumor. Under most circumstances the first step would be to suture the anus closed, which prevents any rectal contents or tumor from spilling out onto the operative field. This was impossible in Penny's situation.

I began by incising the normal appearing skin about two cm from the visible border of the tumor, carrying this incision around the circumference, through the skin and into the subcutaneous fat. And, all I saw was fat. Nothing within the subcutaneous tissues looked like tumor. So far so good. I also was greeted by significant bleeding.

Good and Bad.

Good because the bleeding suggested that the radiation she had received had left the tissue with adequate perfusion. Bad because she lost a significant amount of blood, more than usual for such a procedure. Even so, with a few clamps and the electrocautery, everything was soon under control.

The incision was carried deeper and I began to angle back towards the rectum. I did my best to work smoothly and efficiently, cutting, cauterizing, cutting, clamping, occasionally tying until I was spied the muscle of the levator ani. I started towards the back, first dividing the muscle close to the coccyx, or tailbone, and then dividing it around the rectum. Soon I met up with my dissection from above, entering the pelvis. I brought the rectum down from above, divided the attachments on either side, peeled the rectum off the vagina, and removed the specimen, which I sent off to Pathology for immediate inspection.

I buzzed and clamped a few bleeders and waited.

Maybe I should talk about the weather, ask the scrub tech about her love life. I never know what to talk about while doing nothing.

After the 25-minute eternity, the Pathologist called back.

"Looks good, grossly. Everything appears confined to the skin, maybe a few areas of invasion. I think you're OK on margins."

"Thank you," I replied loudly and then I went back to begin the task of putting Penny back together.

I placed two drains in the pelvis and stitched the levator muscles together.

I hope that will keep any bowel from sinking too far down into the pelvis.

With the rectum gone, the small bowel tends to fill up its space in the pelvis. Years ago, on a different APR and a different patient, the small bowel settled into the pelvis and got stuck. That patient developed a small bowel obstruction about one week after surgery and required a second operation to relieve the obstruction. I hoped to avoid a repeat.

Next, the subcutaneous tissue and skin were closed without difficulty.

That was much easier than I thought it would be.

I changed my gown and gloves and went back to the abdomen. The next order of business was to construct a colostomy. This colostomy would be permanent. I had actually marked the spot where I wanted to put it, checking Penny in upright, sitting, and lying down positions so that the stoma would not sit in a fold, too close to the wound or any bone.

The colostomy completed, the belly was washed out, inspected and closed, and Penny was tucked away in the Recovery Room.

Now it's wait and see how everything heals. I'll keep my fingers and toes crossed.

Why so concerned about healing? One word: Radiation.

Penny's perineum had been treated with full dose radiation and, although it appeared to be healthy with adequate blood supply, one can never be confident with radiated tissue.

And all was well, at least for the first five days. Her colostomy began functioning after a couple of days, she began to eat, and was very stable. I diligently checked the perineal wound each day, looking for any signs of infection or breakdown of the wound.

It started on the sixth day after surgery.

"There's a lot of drainage today," Penny's nurse reported.

Penny's wound began to separate, starting at the back, first a few millimeters, then a centimeter, then ten centimeters, until the entire length of the wound became a gaping hole, exposing the subcutaneous fat, which looked a little grayish.

Penny was started on twice a day dressing changes, I consulted with a Plastic Surgeon, who wasn't very helpful, and contemplated taking her back to surgery to try to close the wound.

Maybe a wound vac will work.

The wound vac is a sponge which is cut to conform to the shape of the open wound, which is then held in place by a clear adhesive. Suction is applied to the sponge. This creates a vacuum which removes any fluid and drainage. The suction also gently pulls the edges of the wound together. The problem with Penny was that the open wound came very close to her vulva.

There doesn't appear to be enough normal skin to get an adequate seal over the wound.

Lack of a seal means that the applied suction won't work, which leaves the wound with just a sponge which becomes a breeding ground for bacteria.

Time to call the wound care specialist.

I called Tom, a very experienced wound care nurse, especially when wound vacs were involved.

"Can't do it," he concluded, "not enough room to get a good seal."

"Thanks for coming, anyway," I answered.

Back to twice a day dressing changes.

And so it went.

Weeks dragged on into months. The wound went from 20 x 15 centimeters, to 18x 14, then 14x10. Then, finally, the open wound had healed enough to allow the wound vac to be placed and Penny's healing accelerated. After four months, it was the size of a fifty-cent piece. At five months, there was just a scab which fell off 3 weeks later. Penny had healed.

I wish I could report that all was well; that the act of trading her anus for a colostomy left her otherwise well. Alas, such was not the case. She still complained of considerable pain and then she popped up with a new lump in her groin.

Her cancer had spread. She began more chemotherapy which did very little. The cancer turned up in her lungs and then her brain. She succumbed to this disease about six months after her wound had finally healed.

I'm not sure I had done her any good.

NIGHT OF THE APPENDIX

It started at 4:30 p.m. Another night on call, only to-day I was covering two busy emergency rooms. It was like that, back in those days, years ago. Our group provided emergency care at four different hospitals and sometimes we covered all of them. Tonight it was two. I wasn't really concerned. There was another surgeon on back-up call and in all the years I'd been in practice there had only been a single episode of simultaneous life threatening emergencies which would have re-quired me to be in two different places at the same time. Luckily, the back-up surgeon came to the rescue in that instance.

But, back to today. This first call from Hospital A was about Lester, 55 years old, with abdominal pain for two days. The pain started in the mid-abdomen and then moved to the right lower quadrant. His white blood cell count was 16,000 and CT Scan of the abdomen and pelvis revealed acute appendicitis.

A no-brainer.

I called the OR and told them to crank up the laparo-scope as I made my way to the ER to see Lester. He was the manager of a well-known used car dealership. His story and exam were textbook, he had an IV, antibiotics were flowing, and the OR crew was ready to take him away.

I commented on the steady beeping of the OR monitors as he drifted off to sleep. The surgery went off without a hitch as I encountered a straightforward, inflamed appendix which I deftly liberated with my trusty Endo GIA stapler, popped into an endopouch, and pulled out in all of 12 minutes.

As I placed the last stitch, my phone went off again. The ER from Hospital B was calling. Dr. P was on the other end of the call.

"I've got a nine-year-old girl with belly pain for four days, temp is 102, and CT shows appendicitis, possibly with an abscess. Do you do kids?"

I answered in the affirmative.

"Does she look very sick?"

"A little flushed, but her heart rate is around a hundred, BP is OK."

"Does she have diffuse tenderness or is it localized?"

"Seems to be confined to the right lower quadrant."

"I think we can do her surgery here. I'll call the OR and I'll be there in a little bit," I informed Dr. P.

I tucked Lester away in the Hospital A PACU, and made the 15-minute drive to Hospital B. It was now 6:15 p.m.

Luisa was a skinny nine-year-old. She smiled at me when I walked in the ER room and winced when I lightly tapped on her RLQ. Her pain had started four days previously, she'd had nausea and vomited about 10 times, and also had diarrhea. Her primary care doctor had diagnosed her with gastroenteritis and prescribed Pedialyte and Bactrim. It's pretty common for appendicitis to be misdiagnosed, delaying evaluation by the surgeon until later in the clinical course. Conditions such as gastroenteritis are very common and, as we are taught in medical school, common things occur commonly. Even though acute appendicitis is one of the most common surgical diseases, acute gastroenteritis is even more common.

Luisa was wheeled off to surgery at 7:12.

She was asleep by 7:35. I put the scope in through her belly button and was greeted by a mass of inflamed bowel and omentum which was oozing pus. It wasn't very attractive and it presented a bit of a challenge. Luisa was not going to be a 12-minute appendectomy.

I started to gingerly dissect. First the omentum. I could see the plane and gently pulled on the tissue. The "watchdog" peeled away so that I could now see a fat, grayish-black appendix nesting against the small bowel, which was my next target. Carefully, carefully, I separated the appendix from the small bowel. A fountain of brownish pus poured out and a large brown "fecalith" rolled down.

"Pac Man," I requested.

The surgical tech rummaged around on her back table and produced the desired instrument, a device which opens and closes its jaws just like the creatures which race around the maze in the Pac Man video game.

I wonder what this instrument's proper name is?

I scooped up the fecalith and whisked it away and deposited it in the basin which was awaiting the offending (and offensive) appendix. Back to the task at hand, I finally had all the bowel and omentum away from the appendix and was able to proceed with what was now a "routine" appendectomy. The appendix was black with a perforation about midway between its tip and the cecum. Luckily the base of the appendix was pink and not involved with the inflammatory process, making the appendectomy straightforward. Once the appendix gone, the final task was irrigating, washing, irrigating and more washing until the peritoneum was clean.

As the final steri strip was placed, my phone chimed again. Hospital A ER was calling.

"This is Dr. T. I've got a 22-year-old male with two days of right lower quadrant abdominal pain, White blood count 22,000, CT shows appendicitis."

Back I went to hospital A. It was now 8:52.

When I arrived in the ER at Hospital A, I met Esteban. He had been having pain for about a day and half. He was lying motionless on the stretcher, his face was slightly flushed. He was thin with a black moustache and he only spoke Spanish.

"Tiene dolor en el estomago?" I asked reaching the limits of my Spanish.

"Si."

"Cuando empezado el dolor?"

And so it went. I can take a reasonable history in Spanish as long as the patient's symptoms are limited to the abdomen and their answers are limited to si or no. Esteban reminded me of one of the rules I learned during residency:

If a young Latino male comes to the ER complaining of right lower quadrant abdominal pain, you can schedule him for appendectomy without seeing him. You will make the proper diagnosis almost one hundred percent of the time.

This was true because it was not considered "macho" to go to the doctor. During residency, back in the 1980's, this rule held true. I'm not so sure being macho is still important. Esteban, however, fell neatly into this category, but he still had been evaluated with the requisite CT Scan which confirmed the obvious diagnosis of acute appendicitis.

He was in the OR by 9:45 and underwent a straight-forward "lap appy," which I finished just in time to get paged to the ER at Hospital B.

"Mary Rogers, 59 years old, right lower abdominal pain for two days, White count is 12,000, CT shows a retrocecal appendicitis," reported the familiar voice of Dr. M.

"Isn't it early for you to call?" I asked Dr. M. "It's usually 2:00 a.m. when I get to hear your voice."

"Be thankful you get an early start tonight," she advised. "Oh and there may be another appendix brewing."

"I'll be there shortly," I answered.

Luckily, the OR crew had not gone home yet. Mary was waiting in the OR holding area when I arrived. I did a quick history and physical, and explained the surgery, and they whisked her away to OR five. It was now 11:10.

The CT Scan was one hundred percent accurate in this case. Mary's appendix was very retrocecal, which means it was hiding behind the cecum (the first part of the colon which is where the appendix is attached), and behind the ascending colon, which is the next part of the colon.

I started by picking up the cecum and identifying the tenia coli, which are bands of muscular tissue in the wall of the colon. There are three tenia on the colon and they meet at the base of the appendix. Following these tenia coli allows the surgeon to find the appendix, which occasionally can be a difficult task. Using this technique I found the base of the appendix, but that was the only portion I could identify. The rest disappeared behind the colon, heading north towards the liver. In order to see what I needed to see, I had to mobilize the right colon, which means divide the peritoneal attachments which keep the colon from flopping around.

This done I now could see the appendix, at least see where it was going. And so I began the tedious, step by step task of clipping the "mesoappendix" which contains the blood vessels going into the appendix. Normally I would take a stapling device and simply divide and staple this mesoappendix with one squeeze, but there was nothing easy about Mary.

Finally, the end was in sight as the inferior edge of the liver came into view. The appendix was inflamed over the distal half, not ruptured, and after much tedious dissection it was finally completely free. Once it was out of the abdomen I measure it at eight inches in length, probably more than twice the norm.

Finally done.

No such luck. The phone went off again.

At least it was Hospital B again. Dr. M greeted me.

"Megan Bartlett is sixteen years old, right lower quadrant abdominal pain for eight hours, White Blood cell count is ten and her CT is normal. She is pretty tender, however."

"OK, I'm still here. I'll come take a look at her," I replied.

Megan was there with two very worried parents, but it soon became obvious that the parents were no longer together and didn't agree on much. Daddy wanted to take his little girl downtown to "World Famous Medical Center." Mommy thought she could stay at Hospital B. I did my usual history and physical exam, reviewed the CT Scan, and then sat down to talk to all the parties involved.

"Megan's history and exam are strongly suggestive of appendicitis," I began, "but the CT looks normal. She's only been sick for eight hours and sometimes the CT won't show any of the usual changes we see with appendicitis if her pain hasn't been going on very long."

I recommended she stay in the hospital to be examined later and if her pain and tenderness persisted, then operate at that time. Mommy was in agreement, but Daddy was still skeptical. I left them alone for a few minutes to hash it out and, in the end, Mommy won out. Daddy was not there when I returned.

Megan was admitted to the Pediatric floor and I went home. It was 2:00 a.m.

I reevaluated Megan in the morning. She was still tender and subsequently underwent an uncomplicated appendectomy.

This night confirmed the old medical adage: "Common things occur commonly."

Appendicitis is one of the most common maladies General Surgeons are called upon to treat. Most of the time this means surgery, although there have been recent efforts made to treat appendicitis nonoperatively with antibiotics. In the end, removal of this offending organ seems to be the best approach. Most patients with uncomplicated appendicitis are discharged within 24 hours and are back to normal activity in a few days.

The advent of CT Scanning to evaluate possible appendicitis has made my life much easier. When I started in the surgery business (too many years ago), the diagnosis and treatment of appendicitis usually took three hours of my time.

Appendicitis was diagnosed based on history, physical exam, and labs. I would drive to the hospital, do my H&P, then call the OR crew, wait for them to arrive and set up, do the surgery, and then go home. Total time: three hours.

Now, the ER physician presents the patient, tells me the CT Scan result, I call the OR crew from home, arrive just before the surgery, perform the operation, and go home. Total time: one hour.

But, I still have to come and evaluate the patient in cases like Megan. Watchful waiting sometimes prevents unnecessary surgery. It is not unusual for the pain to fade away allowing the patient to be discharged without an unnecessary surgical intervention. Often we never find out what caused the pain. Presumably it is a virus or some other self-limiting condition.

Five appendectomies in less than 24 hours is a bit unusual. Recently, I broke this record by doing seven laparoscopic appendectomies in a 24- hour period. Maybe this disease is becoming more common. When I was in medical school, Denis Burkitt, a surgeon who lived in Africa, famous for describing Burkitt's Lymphoma, spoke at one of my classes. He said that appendicitis, among several other diseases like hemorrhoids and colon cancer, was almost never seen in Africa. He chalked it up to America being a "constipated society," one where the highly processed, low fiber diet caused these colonic maladies. I don't know if he is correct. I do know that appendicitis is very common and appears to becoming even more prevalent.

Patients will sometimes ask: "What is the purpose of the appendix?"

I answer: "It gives General Surgeons something to do when we are bored or need to make a car payment."

THE DAY OF THE GALLBLADDERS

It looked like it was going to be a good day. I wasn't on call, I would be off the weekend, and all I had scheduled for the day was four elective cases, all laparoscopic cholecystectomies.

How could the day be any better?

The surgeon's prayer popped into my head:

"Lord, please protect me from the interesting cases and don't let me screw up today."

Cholecystectomy is the most common operation that is performed in the United States. Gallbladder disease occurs as a consequence of diet, hormonal changes, genetics and physiologic changes involving the rest of the body. Everything affects the gallbladder, at least at times it appears that way. Gaining weight, losing weight, pregnancy, illness, stress and probably a whole bunch of other things cause the gallbladder to form stones, stop functioning or become inflamed. Whenever the gallbladder starts to behave badly one can rest assured that a friendly general surgeon is nearby to address the problem.

It was six thirty in the morning, the dogs were fed and I was scheduled to start in an hour.

Maybe I can get rounds done before I surgery.

It was a rare day. I only had patients at one hospital, the same venue where the cases were scheduled. I arrived at six fifty five and greeted my first patient in the Day Surgery Unit.

Maria was 40, about five-foot-one and weighed in at 260 pounds. She had multiple gallstones and had suffered through repeated episodes of right upper quadrant abdominal pain. She had gone to the ER once, but otherwise had endured multiple nights of suffering.

"I just get up and walk around or sit in the chair until the pain goes away, usually after a couple of hours. I take some Motrin, which helps a little."

Textbook case. All Four F's: Female, Fertile, Forty and 'Rotund'.

I went to the hospital computer and checked on each of my in-house patients, their vital signs, lab results, and such. I only had five patients to see. Everyone looked good in the computer.

I suppose I should actually go see each patient.

I ran up to the third floor, the post surgical unit. I saw Bill and Irma and Lucille, each post-op from laparotomies and each was doing well. Notes and orders were written (the good old days, before computerized everything) and then I ran down to the OR to start Maria's surgery.

She was just going to sleep when I walked into OR 5. I went out to wash my hands while she was being prepped.

"Draperies, please," I said.

The tech handed me a towel and I began to drape Maria.

All the proper tools were passed off and connected and surgery commenced.

I infiltrated some long-acting local anesthetic in Maria's belly button area, made a small incision, elevated her abdominal wall, and tried to pass the Veress needle. This needle is what I commonly use to insufflate the abdomen, that is, blow it up with carbon dioxide gas. Only the needle wouldn't reach the peritoneal cavity. I put it in up the hilt, but no go.

She doesn't look to be that large. But, women tend to have their adipose tissue in the abdominal wall. I guess Maria has a bit more than I thought.

"I need a longer Veress needle."

In about a minute, the circulator returned with the 150 cm needle which I was able to pass into the abdomen without difficulty.

I hope that's the only glitch for the day.

And Maria's case went off without a hitch. Inside her abdomen there wasn't much fat. Each structure stood out. The gallbladder was hanging off the liver, the common bile duct was easily seen, and the cystic artery nearly jumped out at me. It was spread, spread, clip, clip, clip, cut, clip, clip, clip, clip, cut, then snip, snip, snip, snoop, and in five minutes the gallbladder was in a pouch, pulled out through the epigastric wound, and on the back table. Ten minutes later the final band-aids were laid over the last of Maria's wounds as she began to wake up. Thirty five minutes after she had gone to sleep, she was in the Recovery Room.

I should have time to see my other two hospital patients.

I saw Joe and Juana on the fourth floor. Neither had a problem which would require surgery. I stopped to say, "Hello, how are you? You should be going home soon." And then went back to the OR to operate on Michael.

Michael had been having pain for years, always in the upper abdomen, radiating to his back, occurring almost every day. He had gone through endoscopies, CT Scans, MRI's, ultrasounds, and more endoscopies. Finally, he found a GI specialist who ordered a HIDA Scan. This is an anatomic and functional test of the gallbladder. In Michael's case, the HIDA revealed his gallbladder only emptied 4% when stimulated and, maybe more important, his symptoms were reproduced... exactly. I told him there was an 85-90% chance his pain would be relieved by surgery.

He was being wheeled into the OR as I finished my rounds.

Should be straightforward. No stones, chronic symptoms, overall in excellent health.

Never make such assumptions.

Michael's surgery started off simple enough. The gallbladder was partially intrahepatic, but that just means a little more dissection until the gallbladder is free. I began in the usual way, incising the thin layer of peritoneum over the neck of the gallbladder and dissecting this peritoneum, and then some surrounding fat away from the wall of the gallbladder. I almost always start on the inferior lateral aspect of the gallbladder, where I should be safely away from the common bile duct.

As I began Michael's dissection, I saw a bluish structure just below the cystic duct and going towards the liver.

Not the right spot for the common bile duct or any bile duct. Be careful. Maybe it will be easier on the other side of the gallbladder.

I began dissecting on the medial aspect of the gallbladder.

It looks like there is another duct on this side. Maybe the gallbladder is lying between the right and left hepatic ducts? The structure in the middle looks like the cystic duct.

I started working higher on the gallbladder, away from any ducts, I hoped.

This is becoming far too much work. This was supposed to be my easy case.

As I dissected along the medial wall of the gallbladder, I was able to identify a duct running along this part of the gallbladder and then going towards the liver. Luckily, I was able to separate this duct from the gallbladder.

That must be the left hepatic duct. At least Michael is not too chunky.

I retracted the gallbladder to the right and began teasing out the cystic duct.

Better check that duct-like structure on the right side of the gallbladder.

It's a good thing I did, because what I thought was all cystic duct turned out to be the right hepatic duct, which was almost fused to the back wall of the gallbladder. I tried to separate these two structures. No luck. I did manage to find what I presumed was the cystic artery, very short and running along the medial aspect of the gallbladder, tethering the gallbladder between the two hepatic ducts.

Maybe take it from the top down, like the old days.

And so I began working on the fundus of the gallbladder. I pushed the liver up and retracted the gallbladder down, and was able to separate the gallbladder until it was attached buy only the cystic duct, which was still fused to the right hepatic duct.

I'll just take where it's safe and leave the rest behind.

I used a stapling device to divide the gallbladder at its neck, being careful not to injure the bile ducts.

Finally done. This was far too much work. I don't think I deserve such aggravation.

Michael woke up without a hitch, oblivious to the torture I had suffered. His operation, which normally would have taken about 30 minutes, had lasted over two hours.

Next was Michelle, 21, with pain for a week and a big stone impacted in the neck of the gallbladder. Michelle was typical of most patients with cholecystitis. That is she had persistent episodes of pain and stones which either intermittently passed from the gallbladder through the bile duct, causing "biliary colic," or had big stones which would cause obstruction of the gallbladder with either acute symptoms of severe pain and tenderness, "acute cholecystitis" or paroxysmal pain, "chronic cholecystitis."

Michael and Michelle, good name for a duo. And now we present, "Michelle and Michael," the gallbladder singers.

My first glance at Michelle's gallbladder revealed only that it was very distended. It wasn't very inflamed and there was only a brief moment when it seemed like there might be some difficulty grasping it. There was a big stone filling the gallbladder neck, but I was able to retract the gallbladder to the right so that I could dissect the cystic artery and duct. 15 minutes later the gallbladder was in the endopouch.

Home free.

But, it wouldn't come out. The pouch was half in and half out of the abdomen, pulling it out through one of the larger trocar sites. I grabbed the gallbladder and tried to deliver it out of the pouch and abdomen. I was rewarded with a tiny piece of the gallbladder wall.

Keep at it. You always win in the end.

I tried to grab the stone with the ring Forceps, a clamp that has two rings, which is ideally suited to grasping gallstones and pulling them out of the Endo-pouch.

Michelle's stone was big, really big. With one lucky swoop I managed to get the jaws of this clamp around the stone. I pulled it up towards the small opening in the abdominal wall. It was equivalent to trying to put a camel through the eye of a needle.

Maybe I can break the stone into little pieces.

I tried to close the jaws of the clamp and break the stone into pieces. There was a "snap" and then I was able to pull the clamp out, minus one of its jaws.

That is one tough stone.

I tried a different type of clamp. No luck.

After twenty minutes of pulling, prying, and hoping, I did what I needed to do.

"Knife, please."

I made the incision bigger, big enough to deliver this baby. I made it bigger and bigger until it was a mini laparotomy. Finally, I pulled pouch, gallbladder, and stone out of Michelle's abdomen.

The stone was five-and-a-half centimeters in diameter, the size of a chicken egg. I took a break for a minute, shaking my hand to relieve a cramp and stretching my fingers after this ordeal. I closed Michelle in short order and got ready for Owen.

I'm definitely sure they don't pay me enough. Maybe Owen will treat me better.

I shouldn't think such thoughts; surely I jinxed myself. Owen. Even now the name makes me shudder. Owen was 78 years old and had typical complaints of RUQ abdominal pain. He had been having pain almost daily for 6 weeks. His ultrasound revealed, and I quote, "Multiple mobile stones," and the gallbladder was not visualized on HIDA Scan, which suggests cystic duct obstruction and certainly explained Owen's frequent symptoms.

"Are you ready to get this over with?" I asked.

"Sure thing, Doc. I'm planning to play 18 holes tomorrow," He answered.

"Well, you may want to wait until the weekend," I countered.

Owen's case started well enough. Pneumoperitoneum established without difficulty, all the trocars placed and then I looked in with the scope.

No gallbladder.

All I saw was a bit of omentum stuck to the spot where the gallbladder was supposed to be.

It must be underneath those adhesions.

I teased the omentum away and was rewarded with a structure that looked like it was the gallbladder. It was small to say the least, but it was where the gallbladder was supposed to sit and I was sure I could see the common bile duct.

Once the adhesions were gone, I began to retract the gallbladder superiorly as is almost always done during laparoscopic gallbladder surgery. The gallbladder was not only shrunken, it was very hard to grasp. Every time I tried to grab it, it would slip away. Finally, all I could do was push the liver superiorly. As I tried to dissect this diminutive little beast, it tore. I did see some stones inside but I realized I was fighting a losing battle.

"Scalpel, please, and get all the instruments to open," I requested.

Better to have a big incision and a healthy, whole patient, than four small incisions and a piece of the common bile duct in the specimen jar.

Over the years I have never had a patient complain that they had to have open surgery. However, they definitely are not happy if they require multiple surgeries to fix a transected common bile duct.

For the next hour and a half I wrestled with Owen's little nubbin of a gallbladder. I managed to separate it from the liver and I thought I found his cystic duct and junction with the common bile duct. The cystic duct was very short. I stitched it closed, being careful not to narrow his CBD, and I left a drain in place.

I delivered a gallbladder that was the size of a nickel and contained a couple of stones that filled its tiny lumen.

Two hours of work for that little thing?

Owen woke up without a hitch.

"No golf for a few weeks," I informed him.

"There goes my handicap," he answered.

At least I'm done.

My phone went off.

"Consult, ICU 21. Tad Schultz, acute cholecystitis."

I thought I was done.

It was now 3:30 in the afternoon. My plan to be done and home by 1:00 p.m. was just a fading memory.

I guess I need to go check out Tad. I wonder why he's in ICU if it's just his gallbladder that is the problem?

Tad was not in the ICU just because of his gallbladder. He had undergone coronary artery bypass surgery 36 hours ago. Now he was complaining of severe upper abdominal pain, nausea, and vomiting, all of which had commenced 12 hours earlier.

"Hello, Mr. Schultz. I'm Dr. Gelber, one of the General Surgeons here. They tell me you have pain in your abdomen?" I inquired.

He was sitting still in his bed, an oxygen cannula draped across his face which was flushed. The monitor to the right of his bed gave a clue to his condition. Heart rate was 112, blood pressure 100/50, Respirations 22, oxygen saturation was 100%.

Looks like something is going on; something more than just post-op discomfort.

"It hurts right here," he replied as he pointed to the right upper quadrant of his abdomen, right where his gallbladder sat. "It hurts to move, to breath, even to smile," he added.

I wonder if it's more than just his gallbladder?

"Any nausea or vomiting?"

"All night."

"Had a pain like this before?"

"Never."

I palpated his abdomen. He winced when I lightly tapped beneath the right costal margin (below the ribs).

It feels like there's a mass there.

"I'll be back in a few minutes," I said and I went to check the results of any testing that had been done.

I sat at the computer, waiting for Tad's data to appear.

I don't feel like doing another surgery today, especially on someone fresh from open-heart surgery.

The tests revealed that his White Blood Cell count was 23,000, H/H 10.5 and 32. Total bilirubin was 2.0, ALT 125, AST 114, and Alkaline Phosphatase 201. His other labs were more or less normal. Ultrasound revealed a very distended gallbladder with stones and a thickened wall at 10 mm.

No question, Tad is sick and the culprit is his gall-bladder. Fresh from open heart surgery, another operation so soon would best be avoided, if possible. Maybe Dr. L can help.

Dr. L was our local, friendly, always willing to help Interventional Radiologist.

"Percutaneous cholecystostomy, if you have the time," I requested from Dr. L. "Mr. Schultz, ICU 21. I think it would be best if he does not have to have surgery again so soon."

Instead of a second major operation, Tad would have a drainage tube placed into his gallbladder by Dr. L. I hoped.

Dr. L agreed and two hours later Tad was sitting up, smiling, with a tube running from his right flank to a bag that was filled with golden brown bile.

It was not definitive treatment, but the drainage procedure bought time, allowing Tad to recover from his open-heart surgery without further complication. Six weeks later he had a second surgery, an uncomplicated laparoscopic cholecystectomy.

The day ended at around 6:00 pm. I had performed four cholecystectomies, tackling gallbladders of a variety of shapes and complexities. My hand was still a little sore from battling Michelle's ostrich egg of a gallstone, but otherwise it had been a successful day.

Cholecystectomy can be one of the easiest surgeries to perform or extremely difficult. An elective gallbladder surgery in a thin patient with little inflammation and normal anatomy may take all of 10 minutes. Meanwhile, at the other end of the spectrum, a case like Owen, a small contracted, fibrotic gallbladder with anatomy which is unclear, will cause the best surgeon to pause and rue the day he chose to work with a scalpel, rather than sit in a dark room all day and read chest X-Rays. I thought about the surgeon's prayer again:

"Lord, please protect me from the interesting cases and don't let me screw up today."

Maybe it needs an addendum:

"And please make all the gallbladder surgeries easy."

TO CUT IS TO CURE

The title above is an old medical saying which means: "The act of performing surgery often cures a patient from whatever condition is ailing him or her."

This contrasts with "medical" management which is the way of treatment for many chronic medical conditions such as Congestive Heart Failure, Diabetes, Hypertension, and so many others. These conditions are treated primarily with pills and lifestyle changes, surgery being reserved for complications of the underlying illness. Such diseases are managed, not cured. Examples of such surgery are joint replacement in the severe arthritic or amputation of a limb as a complication of Diabetes. These operations relieve symptoms and can be lifesaving, but the underlying disease is not cured.

There are, however, many instances where surgery is truly curative. Appendicitis comes to mind. The inflamed appendix is removed and the patient is never troubled by appendicitis again.

Then there are instances where a patient has suffered for years, seen a multitude of doctors, and been treated with pills, surgery, and everything else, but continues to suffer. It seems like nothing will provide relief. Even so, such patients grasp at the narrowest of straws, hoping against hope that surgery, i.e. "to cut," will lead to a cure. Patricia was such a patient.

She was 37 years old and I was asked to see her for small bowel obstruction. She had previously undergone 12 abdominal surgeries which included a subtotal gastrectomy for a "lazy stomach" (a condition called gastroparesis), cholecystectomy, hysterectomy, appendectomy, and multiple operations for small bowel obstruction.

The records indicated that over the prior 18 months she had been operated on five times for small bowel obstruction, four by the same surgeon. Each time the procedure was "lysis of adhesions" which means cutting away scar tissue. And, each time she would feel better for a short time, but her symptoms always returned.

She had become dependent on pain medication, taking narcotics on a daily basis. Her abdomen had scars running up and down and crossways. Her imaging studies looked like a classic small bowel obstruction, dilated small bowel transitioning to collapsed bowel. However, her post gastrectomy reconstruction was with a Roux-en-Y gastrojejunostomy, which is common after most of the stomach has been removed. This type of reconstruction can alter the normal appearance of the small bowel on X-Rays.

The Roux Y loop of bowel which is connected to the stomach often dilates as it assumes some of the role of the stomach. Thus, this dilated small bowel often is interpreted as small bowel obstruction, rather than the consequence of the physiologic change associated with its new function of replacing the portion of stomach that has been surgically removed.

Patricia reported nausea and vomiting, and she said the emesis was bilious fluid which is very uncommon after Roux-en-Y reconstruction. She also reported passing flatus and having regular bowel movements which suggested she was not completely obstructed.

Gathering all the information together, I elected not to operate on her initially. She was managed with a nasogastric tube and gradually improved so that she could eat and she was sent home. She returned three weeks later with the exact same symptoms and X-Ray findings.

She'll probably need another surgery.

Before plunging back into what I was sure would be a very difficult surgical exploration, more workup was called for. Upper GI endoscopy revealed a very small gastric pouch, some gastritis, but nothing to explain her X-Ray findings. UGI series was done and these X-Rays corroborated the CT Scan findings of incomplete small bowel obstruction. The ingested contrast did pass all the way through, the proximal bowel was dilated, and there was no discernible stricture.

Maybe I should watch her a bit longer, maybe she'll open up. Maybe it's all related to her narcotic use.

So I watched and waited, and she didn't get better.

No choice. Operation number 13 coming up.

I did have a plan of sorts. As best as I could determine, she always presented with a dilation of her Roux-en-Y limb which was connected to her stomach, and then the bowel became normal a short distance beyond.

There must be an adhesion or stricture in that area.

The big day came. She looked up at me in the moments before she went to sleep with a look of hope in her eyes.

I wonder if her previous surgeons had seen that same look.

I made a midline incision and gingerly worked my way into her abdomen. I managed to get into the peritoneal cavity without causing any serious damage. The adhesions were not nearly as nasty as I'd encountered in other patients, at least not yet.

I cut my way through the web of scar tissue which was encrusting some normal caliber small bowel, suggesting that this bowel was downstream from the real problem area. As I made my way towards the small bowel's beginnings, the adhesions became denser and I soon encountered a very dilated loop of small intestine. This told me I was at least getting close to an area where her pathology might be found.

After a while I reached a point where the scar tissue was extremely dense. Usually when I encounter something like this, I will change direction. Look for another angle or approach that might make the task simpler. I began my assault on the adhesions at a different point, an easier point, and at first I was rewarded.

I figured out that I was dissecting the Roux-en-Y limb and that this would lead to what was left of her stomach. This loop of bowel was very dilated suggesting that it was obstructed. After a bit more careful snipping, I struck gold (or was it oil?). Anyway, I found where two segments of small bowel had been anastomosed (connected together), and a point where the dilated bowel collapsed to normal caliber. This was just beyond the point where the bowel coming from the stomach was reconnected to the rest of the small bowel. There were extensive adhesions here, and my first thought was that cutting away this scar tissue would solve poor Patricia's problem.

In the course of my dissection, I made a new assault on the area of dilated small bowel involved with the densest adhesions, and was able to discern that this was a segment of bowel which originated at her duodenum. It was also very dilated. So, I had two limbs of small bowel which were both dilated. Both remained dilated up to the point where they were connected, but just beyond this area the small bowel was normal. I had lysed the very dense adhesions encasing these loops of bowel and they were now completely free.

Could it be that simple?

It was at this point I either was very smart or very lucky. In the course of my dissection, I had inadvertently made a hole in the small bowel. (Nobody's perfect.)

This hole was just beyond the point of obstruction. Palpation of the area did not suggest anything particularly unusual. The anastomosis from her previous surgery looked and felt wide open and the bowel itself felt soft, rather than fibrotic. But, I decided to put my finger inside the bowel. After all, I already had a hole in the bowel.

Much to my surprise and relief, there was a definite stricture, a ring of hard, fibrotic tissue which narrowed the bowel to about 1/4 its normal caliber. And there was no question that this was the point of obstruction; this was where the dilated bowel collapsed to normal.

This is her problem. But how to fix it?

It really didn't take much thought. I could have redone the entire Roux-en-Y limb, which would have involved taking all the previous connections apart and starting over. Or, I could do a stricturoplasty, which would means doing something at the point of the stricture to widen it. This probably would have worked, but I worried that it could restricture and then Patricia would be back where she started.

I decide to let physics rule the day and bypass around the stricture. Physics comes into play because fluid passing through a tube will tend to take the path of least resistance. In Patricia's case, the fluid which now originated in the duodenum, which is composed of bile from the liver and pancreatic juices, was, for the most part, taking the path of least resistance, which was up the Roux-en-Y limb to her stomach instead of downstream through the rest of her small bowel. Creating a new outlet for the Roux-en-Y limb should provide relief. Therefore, I took the simple, easy way out and connected the Roux-en-Y limb, which was attached to her stomach, to the small bowel beyond the stricture. This allowed food from the stomach to avoid the stricture and the duodenal fluid to go around the stricture also, passing briefly into the Roux-en-Y limb, but then exiting via the newly created outlet.

This task completed, I made a graceful exit form Patricia's abdomen and then sat back and waited. The first morning after surgery I was greeted by a definite absence of bile draining from her NG tube. And she noticed a difference immediately. She sailed through an uneventful post-op course and was discharged home after about a week, eating a regular diet.

On her post-op visit in the office, she had gained four pounds and she made this comment:

"For the first time in seven years I don't wake up with the taste of bile in my mouth."

She has continued to heal uneventfully.

Truly, "To cut is to cure," but sometimes it helps to be lucky.

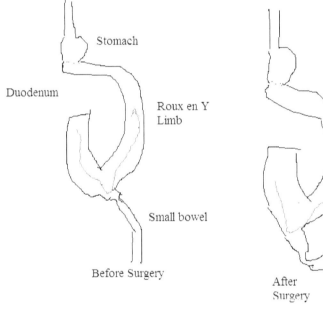

Stomach

Duodenum

Roux en Y
Limb

Small bowel

Before Surgery

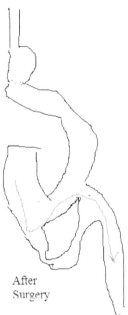

After
Surgery

WORRY

I've been practicing as a general surgeon for 25 years, more or less. All these years have taught me many things, but there is one thing I've learned to do very well: worry.

As a general surgeon I take care of very sick patients. I perform complicated operations on severely injured or septic people and care for them afterwards, watching for any little sign that may be the harbinger of something worse to come.

So, I worry.

I worry about wounds healing, anastomoses leaking, infections brewing, blood clots forming, and a variety of other events which can and do occur after surgery.

A case-in-point is Denny.

Denny was a young man who came to be my patient one night when I was on call for the emergency room. He had been stabbed eight years before I saw him and had sported a colostomy ever since that event. I guess he finally became tired of having a bag, because he had undergone a colonoscopy earlier that day in anticipation of having his colostomy reversed. Unfortunately, he developed severe pain after his colonoscopy.

Despite his protests to the endoscopist that he was in pain, he was sent home. He returned to the ER, at a different facility from where his colonoscopy had been performed, where the work up revealed he had free intraperitoneal air, which meant his colon had been perforated during the colonoscopy.

Denny refused to go back to the hospital where the colonoscopy had been done and so I took him to surgery. I found that his colon had perforated at the splenic flexure, an area that was "defunctionalized," which means that his colostomy was proximal to this injured segment of colon.

The perforation was at the closed off "blind pouch." There was essentially no fecal contamination and all that was required was to close the perforation. I did examine the rest of his colon and even contemplated reversing the colostomy at that time, but properly decided not to. I wasn't privy to the findings from the colonoscopy, and emergency surgery would not be considered optimal conditions to perform such a procedure. I did leave the blind end sutured to the segment of colon where the colostomy was so that subsequent reversal would be easier to perform. At least, that was my plan.

No real worries up to this point, but Denny's troubles were just beginning.

He recovered uneventfully from this procedure and went home after about five days. During his post-op visit he asked about reversing the colostomy.

"Sure," I replied, "once you've healed enough from this surgery. I did leave the two ends of the colon together so that the reversal should be easier."

He was happy with this answer. I sent him on his way with a follow-up appointment for a month later and instructions to "take it easy" until I saw him again.

Well, he missed his next appointment. I assumed he was recovering adequately since I had not heard from him. My office staff made their usual effort to contact him and found out his phone was disconnected. He had been well at the last visit so I wasn't very concerned.

Two weeks later I was called from the ER where Denny had made a return visit complaining of abdominal pain.

"Denny's CT reveals some inflammation around his colon and Dr. M wants you to consult," the ER physician reported.

"Sure," I replied. "Is Denny stable?"

"Just left-sided abdominal pain, otherwise he's fine."

I saw him later in the day and he was already feeling better. He quickly recovered and we made plans for him to have his colostomy reversed in about six weeks. He had pre-op evaluation with a barium enema. His recent colonoscopy had revealed only a bit of diverticulosis, which the barium enema confirmed.

He underwent a fairly uneventful reversal of his colostomy. There was a little bit of excitement as the distal colon which I had sutured adjacent to the colostomy was not where I had left it, but a bit of searching identified the wayward bowel and he sailed through his recovery and went home.

But, not for long.

Two months later I was called to the ER. Denny was there and complaining of lower abdominal pain.

"CT looks like sigmoid diverticulitis with a small abscess," reported the ER doc. "He looks pretty stable. The hospitalist is admitting him and he's consulted you."

"OK, thanks," I answered. "I'll see him when I'm done in surgery."

Denny didn't look very ill and I fully expected his diverticulitis to resolve with only IV antibiotics. At first the plan worked. His pain improved, his low-grade fever improved, and his elevated WBC came down to nearly normal. But, after three days, his condition changed. He developed fever and his WBC went back up. I repeated his CT scan and it revealed a new, larger abscess.

I made a call to Interventional Radiology. The abscess was drained and he settled down again... for a while. He continued to drain and then developed new onset of fever and abdominal pain. He had developed a second abscess. It was fast becoming apparent that he was headed to surgery again.

He was not so sick, however, that I needed to rush him to the Operating Room. Time was taken to drain the new abscess and properly prepare him for what I suspected was going to be a major undertaking. After a few more days of antibiotics, bowel preparation, and soul searching, his time arrived.

The operation was not what I expected. He had a few adhesions which were easily dispatched. The inflamed segment of colon was mid-sigmoid, there was plenty of uninvolved proximal and distal colon.

Not nearly as bad as expected.

The time for worrying had not yet arrived.

I resected the inflamed segment of colon and prepared to do the anastomosis, that is, to reconnect the two ends of the pipe, when I took a closer look at the bowel.

Is the blood supply to the proximal segment adequate?

Normally, I wouldn't think twice about this. The surgery was for benign disease which means most of the blood supply is left intact. But something about Denny made me pause and think twice. He had undergone several previous colon operations which almost certainly caused some sort of alteration to the normal blood supply.

The bowel did appear healthy and adequately perfused. I could see arteries in the mesentery which were
intact and I even thought I could feel a pulse.

Perhaps check it with a Doppler? Better safe than
sorry.

Unfortunately, this was not very helpful. The Doppler is a sort of ultrasound that detects flow in blood
vessels. In Denny's case there was definitely arterial
blood flow in the mesentery, but I did not hear it very
well in the bowel.

Perhaps it would be best to resect more colon?

To remove more bowel would leave him with very
little colon as I would be forced to remove the previous
anastomosis and then there would be difficulty reconnecting the two ends.

What to do? Go with my gut?

I hate that expression.

Reason and experience told me that doing the anastomosis without removing any additional bowel would
be OK, and so I proceeded.

And the worry started, also.

Perhaps it is a part of growing older and wiser, but I
worry much more now than when I first started out as a
surgeon. We were always taught to not take chances, to
be sure of what was being done or else pursue an alter-
nate course, one that would eliminate uncertainty.

"If it's not safe to do an anastomosis, do a colostomy. Better a live patient with a colostomy, than a dead
patient," my mentors said.

"If you're not sure if it's the cystic duct or common
bile duct, don't assume, don't cut it, don't do anything
until you are sure," another instructor bellowed.

"See the nerve, see the nerve," a third teacher commanded.

But what about those times when the operative course is not cut and dry?

Do it this way and the patient should be fine, unless this happens. But if I do it the other way, then this could happen.

Denny presented several options, each with positives and negatives:

1. Do the planned procedure, the resection and anastomosis, and presume it will heal.

2. Extend the resection which will leave him with a very short colon, but less worry about healing.
3. Do the planned procedure, but add a proximal colostomy or ileostomy. The proximal diversion of the fecal stream would allow the colon anastomosis to heal and then the ostomy could be closed in a few months.

There were plusses and minuses for each alternative. Number one was best for Denny, assuming he healed properly. No further surgery needed, fewer long-term complications such as frequent diarrhea associated with a short colon.

There would be little worrying with Number Two as the blood supply would not be in question and healing should proceed with little risk of anastamotic breakdown, but he would likely be troubled by very frequent bowel movements.

Number Three might be best as it preserved his colon, but would require another operation down the road to reverse the colostomy or ileostomy.

What to do? What to do?

In the end I decided on Number One, my original plan. I decided the colon had adequate blood supply, had been properly prepped, and, if everything healed properly, would be best for Denny.

But it didn't stop me from worrying.

What does this worrying entail?

That night I called to check on his condition. Normally I check on my ICU patients, but Denny did not need to be in the unit.

His heart rate was a tad high at 110, but everything else was fine: good urine output, no fever, no unusual pain. I didn't really expect any issues immediately post surgery. His issues, should they develop, would become manifest in 4 days or 10 days or 2 weeks.

So, I waited and checked and waited. I carefully palpated his abdomen on daily rounds, looking for any tenderness that was greater than expected. I looked at his heart rate, coming down from 110 to 104 to 95, and my confidence rose as it dropped.

Tachycardia is the first sign that something is amiss.

The first wisp of flatus almost brought cheers as his bowel function returned to normal. By the fourth day after surgery everything was normal: white blood cell count, heart rate, kidney function. He was tolerating a liquid diet and his bowel function was normal.

In addition, my heart rate, blood pressure, and everything else was normal.

Denny went on to an uneventful recovery and is back to normal.

Was my worry warranted, productive, or unnecessary? Shouldn't I be as vigilant and worry about every patient?

The vast majority of the surgery I do is cut and dry. Right upper quadrant abdominal pain with gallstones? Take out the gallbladder.

Malignant tumor in the cecum? Take out that part of the colon.

Single hyper-functioning parathyroid gland causing severely elevated calcium level? Take out the offending gland.

Straightforward cases such as these, performed properly, usually have uncomplicated postoperative courses and rarely cause me to lose any sleep, except when they do. I always maintain a watchful eye, but complications in well-planned and well-executed surgeries rarely rear their ugly head.

But cases like Denny, where the proper course is not as clearly defined, are different. Suppose he had leaked from his anastomosis. Or suppose I had taken a different course, removed more colon, and he developed intractable diarrhea. Or suppose I had taken the intermediate course and he developed a pulmonary embolus and died during the surgery to reverse his ostomy.

Worrying about complicated cases goes with the turf of being a physician. In the end, all one can do is look back and say: "I looked at all the possibilities and chose the best option. If the same situation arises again, I'll do the same thing. Worrying doesn't help."

But, the little nagging pest named worry still whispers in my ear.

AMAZING CASE

Over the many years I've been trying to perfect the art of surgery, I've been involved with some truly interesting and amazing surgeries. By far, those cases that pique my interest the most are the retroperitoneal tumors.

I don't know if it's the challenge of having to navigate my way around an array of anatomic structures bearing names that were learned in elementary school, such as aorta, kidney, and pancreas, or the satisfaction that comes from knowing that successfully performing these operations gives the patient hope, or if it's the joy of performing a truly anatomic dissection. But these are some of my favorite cases.

I know that I may face rebuke from my half a dozen fans for making such a statement, one which directly contradicts the Surgeon's Prayer: "Lord, protect me from the interesting cases…," but there is still a bit of the adventurous surgeon inside of me.

What is the Retroperitoneum? As the name implies, it is the part of the abdomen which is retro, or behind, the peritoneum. The peritoneum is the thin membrane which covers much of our intraabdominal viscera or organs. The stomach, most of our intestines, the liver, and spleen all lay within the peritoneal cavity.

252 | *Amazing Days, Endless Nights*

Behind this cavity, in the back of the abdomen, are the organs and blood vessels of the retroperitoneum. The pancreas, kidneys, ureters, adrenal glands, aorta, and inferior vena cava are the retroperitoneum's major structures; organs and blood vessels surgeons have learned should be accorded the utmost respect and avoided if at all possible.

"Stay away from the Pancreas," barked Dr. F.

"Find the Ureter," commanded Dr. D.

"Be careful of the Vena Cava," warned Dr. B.

I must have a masochistic bent to welcome potential calamity into my OR suite.

Eulie came to the office one day. She was 68, in reasonably good health, only mild hypertension and had vague complaints of abdominal pain. She bore with her reports of her recent CT Scan of her abdomen and pelvis.

"Occlusion of the Inferior Vena Cava by thrombus or tumor 7.4 cm in length, starting above the renal veins and extending to below the confluence of the hepatic veins. Comparison with CT Scan performed on May 23, 2014, reveals the intraluminal mass has increased from 3.8 cm to its present size. Minimal flow is noted within the vena cava. Renal veins appear patent."

Eulie had never had any symptoms suggestive of acute occlusion of the IVC and my first impression was that this was a tumor. Her physical exam was unremarkable.

"I think you are going to need surgery to remove what looks like a tumor in the Inferior Vena Cava," I recommended. "I need to go over to the hospital to look at the actual images."

The scope and intricate nature of the proposed surgery were explained and she left, surgery tentatively planned for two weeks hence.

"It looks like a tumor growing in the vena cava," I commented as I scanned the recent CT Scan.

Dr. L, an exceptional radiologist, agreed.

"It looks like you should have a good cuff of Vena Cava below the hepatic veins to work with," he observed.

"Yes, but I hope I'll just have to ligate it. It looks like it's been pretty much occluded for a year," I replied, alluding to the scan from last year.

"Let me know what you find," Dr. L requested as I walked away.

I put Eulie out of my mind for the time being as I had plenty of other sick people to occupy my time.

10 days later, Eulie popped up again as her name appeared on my schedule for the following day. She was booked to follow two cholecystectomies on two other patients.

The next morning I removed the two gallbladders in workmanlike fashion, these two cases acting as warm ups for Eulie's far more complicated surgery.

I made my usual pre-op visit to her and said hello to the large contingent of family and friends who would be waiting on her, then I went off to make rounds on a few patients while the staff prepared the operating room.

At 9:28 a.m. Eulie was wheeled back to the OR, moved from stretcher to OR table, and in less than 10 minutes was asleep. The operation still had to wait while anesthesia personnel placed a central line, arterial line, and the nurse placed a urinary catheter and cleansed her abdomen with the antiseptic solution: Chloraprep.

Finally they were ready for me. But first the time out:

"Eulie ___, 68, DOB ___, she's scheduled for resection of Vena Cava tumor, no allergies…"

254 | *Amazing Days, Endless Nights*

I mumbled my agreement and we commenced.

I started with a long midline incision from xiphoid, which is the lower end of the breastbone, to just above the pubis.

A real operation for a change. No scopes, no monitors.

I really don't have anything against minimally invasive surgery. Laparoscopic, thoracoscopic, and endovascular approaches are much better for the patient. But there is something about getting your hands into the patient, actually feeling the organs, normal and pathologic, that adds a dimension to the surgery that is almost completely lost with laparoscopic approaches and absolutely absent from robotic surgery.

The firmness of the liver contrasting with the soft suppleness of normal bowel, the pulses of major arteries and the hardness of malignant tumors cannot be fully appreciated by the limited sense of touch transmitted through long laparoscopic instruments.

William Halsted, the founder of the department of Surgery at Johns Hopkins Hospital, eschewed the use of gloves because he did not want to lose the tactile sense he had with his bare hand. Bare-handed surgery seems barbaric now, but back in those days, the first rubber gloves were made for Dr. Halsted's nurse, not for sterility. No, they were developed because her hands were sensitive to the mercuric chloride and carbolic acid used as antiseptics during surgery at that time. I wonder what Dr. Halsted would say now as we have almost given up the sense of touch during surgery. Progress?

Back to Eulie's operation.

At first nothing unusual was seen in Eulie's abdomen. No free fluid, no immediate signs of malignancy, just normal liver, stomach, and bowel. I ran my hand over the presumed area of the Inferior Vena Cava and everything was soft, at first. But then, as I palpated the area of the porta hepatis, there was something hard behind the bile duct, portal vein, and duodenum.

Time to start the surgery.

First step is mobilization and exposure. There were several layers of organs between me and the Inferior Vena Cava. First is the colon and omentum. Cut on the dotted line and bring the colon and omentum from right to left, and five minutes later it's out of my way, leaving the duodenum, porta hepatis, and part of the pancreas to contend with.

Mobilizing these structures starts with a Kocher maneuver, named for surgeon of old, Emil Theodor Kocher. The attachments of the duodenum to the retroperitoneum are divided which allows me to lift the duodenum and the head of the pancreas off the Inferior Vena Cava, leaving Big Blue (as the IVC is affectionately called by me) exposed.

At this point it is apparent that the mass in the IVC is not a clot; it is most definitely a tumor. The renal veins and aorta are also exposed. The tumor extends well into the retrohapatic cava. Proximal control will require a different approach.

I turn my attention to the IVC which is adjacent to the caudate lobe of the liver. This part of the IVC is one I usually wave at while doing hiatal hernia surgery, as it is adjacent to the esophageal hiatus, which is where the esophagus passes through the diaphragm. Normally, I try to avoid any contact with it.

More mobilization, this time division of the lesser omentum and retraction of the left lobe of the liver and caudate lobe, and the IVC is exposed again, this time almost behind the liver, but just above the tumor. Dissection of the vena cava even more proximally proved to be dicey as Big Blue took a dive towards the back. There was adequate vena cava to clamp above the tumor but reconstruction, if necessary, would be a bit more problematic.

The final part of the dissection was to lift the porta hepatis off the vena cava and tumor. The porta consists of the extrahepatic bile ducts, hepatic artery and portal vein, all vital structures. Once again, the surgery gods shined their faces upon me as the porta hepatis was easily dissected free and retracted away from the cava.

And, there we were, me and the vena cava and the tumor, staring at each other. A moment of truth had been reached. The real operation was about to commence.

Clamp…clamp…cut? No.

Dissect a bit more, perhaps. Mobilize the tumor away from the aorta and free it from the tissue behind.

Easy… No problem.

Now, do a bit of work around the kidneys, where there might be a bit of a problem. The Left Renal Vein comes in to the cava right above the lower end of the tumor, while the Right Renal Vein right enters below the left. There is no way I can properly resect the tumor without doing something with the renal veins.

Left Renal Vein is no problem. Ligate it and all should be well. This vein can drain through the gonadal and adrenal veins which branch off the left renal. These branches provide adequate collateral flow for the Left Renal Vein.

But the Right Renal Vein is an issue.

I'll have to re-implant it somehow. I'll deal with it later. Time to get the tumor out.

I started with the Ligasure, a marvelous device that seals and cuts blood vessels. This Ligasure eliminates the old clamp, clamp, cut, and tie, reducing a three-minute maneuver to ten or fifteen seconds.

As I buzzed away, very efficiently I must say, I was forced to pause as blood started squirting at me, bright red, arterial blood. Suction was applied followed by my finger, right over the aorta. It seems my wonderful Ligasure was not very competent at sealing this particular vessel. Oh well, a bit of old-fashioned halstedian surgery is good for the soul. I called for 4-0 Prolene and the small artery arising from the aorta was sutured with minimal fuss.

Was it just a minor annoyance? Or, a bit of ominous foreshadowing?

I continued on with my dissection until the vena cava and the tumor were completely free, both renal veins were dissected, and I had adequate vena cava above and below the tumor to, at least, ligate.

The moment of truth had arrived.

The Left Renal Vein was clamped and divided, then the Right Renal Vein, followed by the retrohepatic cava. This vessel was clamped without any change in Eulie's vital signs, and then the vena cava below the tumor was clamped, once again with no change in vital signs. Finally the vena cava itself was divided above and below the tumor, which was removed and sent off to the waiting arms of the Pathologist for her gentle perusal.

Home free? But where's that blood coming from?

There was dark blood welling up adjacent to the liver from the area of the proximal clamp.

Suck… suck…

Just great, there's a tear in the vena cava above the clamp.

"I need another vascular clamp," I announced, hoping the tech was paying attention. "A straight clamp."

Carefully, carefully, I slip the clamp on the cava above the area which is bleeding, and the pool of blood disappears into the suction, banished forever I hope.

Doesn't look like enough to sew. Maybe I can slide the clamp a few millimeters higher?

With as much care as I can muster, I loosen the clamp enough to move it closer to the heart. This leaves me with about 5 millimeters of vena cava to work with. Plenty to ligate, but not enough to sew a graft.

OK, ligation should be good enough. The cava's been completely occluded for at least a year anyway.

"4-0 Prolene, please," I request and then I stick out my hand.

The suture appears, not rudely slapped into my palm, like TV or the movies, more gracefully, gently.

"I've never done a case like this," the tech announces. "Is this like an aortic aneurysm."

"Yes, only more so," I answer.

Worse, much worse. If that clamp comes off before I finish sewing then poor Eulie will be dead.

Think of having a big hole in the bottom of the heart.

But, it doesn't come off, the cava is ligated successfully and I can finally breathe.

What next? The Right Renal Vein.

It won't reach the cava. I guess I'll need to make Big Blue a bit bigger. There is also a large lumbar vein which I've preserved, much larger than normal, which suggests it may have been acting as an important collateral vessel.

"I need a graft, looks like a 20 mm Hemashield Platinum will work," I announce, hoping the circulator is listening.

She is right on top of things; the graft is already in the room.

With minimal fuss, I suture the graft to the clamped Vena Cava, and re-implant the renal vein and the lumbar vein. The moment of truth arrives, the clamp is released, and voila, everything looks good.

Specifically, Eulie has normal vital signs and there's no bleeding anywhere. The Pathologist reports back and says the tumor looks like a sarcoma, the caval margins are free of tumor, but the cancer does extend to the radial margin, which means it has grown through the wall of the vena cava.

Nothing else to do. The duodenum was up against the tumor. The risk of resecting this far outweigh potential benefits.

"Number one PDS to close, please."

And so it went.

Eulie's recovery was marred by a brief episode of hypotension, which responded to IV fluids and a couple of units of blood. She had a transient rise in BUN and Creatinine, but these rapidly returned to baseline and she was home in five days.

Eulie was a case of knowing what is and what is not possible. The Left Renal Vein has collateral vessels which allow it to be ligated safely. The Right Renal Vein is not as forgiving. The Inferior Vena Cava lies deep within the retroperitoneum.

Proper knowledge of how to expose and work around Big Blue should be a part of every general surgeon's training. It is a vessel that can be most unforgiving if injured; sometimes trying to sew it is akin to putting stitches in wet tissue paper. Happily, this was not the case with Eulie.

Complex surgery, like Eulie's, requires some planning and forethought. What I mean by this is that after all the preoperative evaluation; the history, physical, blood tests, and imaging is done, the plan for the actual operation needs development.

What incision is best?

How best to expose and control the vena cava?

Will anything need to be done with kidneys or their major vessels?

Will the vena cava need reconstruction or simple ligation?

These and other questions were mulled over again and again as I tried to anticipate each and every possibility. In Eulie's case, all my planning led to a successful operation and outcome.

A few days after the surgery, the Oncologist on the case stopped me.

"I read your operative note. I'll bet your heart was racing during much of Eulie's surgery," he commented.

"No, just all in a day's work," I lied.

We both smiled.

BATTLE OF THE BOWELS

It was Friday afternoon and I was on call for the weekend. Dr. A from the ER was on the other end of the phone.

I really don't feel like working.

"I've got a good case for you," she began. "Mickey M., 45, no medical problems, has had abdominal pain for four days, and CT shows a large amount of free intraperitoneal air."

"Is he stable?" I asked.

"Vital signs are normal, no fever, white count is 18,000, but…"

There's always a "but."

"…he weighs 410 pounds."

"Okay," I sighed, "I'll be there to see him shortly."

A good case?

I called the OR and scheduled him for surgery, and then walked across the street to make a proper assessment of Mickey.

At least he had the courtesy to come in at 1:30 in the afternoon instead of midnight.

Mickey was large in every sense of the word. He was six-foot-three, his belly was almost as tall as he lay on the ER stretcher, his face was flushed, and he was a little sweaty and a more than a little short of breath.

His numbers didn't look that bad: heart rate 90, blood pressure 145/85, respirations 24, oxygen saturation 97% on room air, temperature normal. He had never had previous surgery, took no medications. He winced when I tapped his abdomen.

Besides the elevated white blood count, he was anemic with a hemoglobin of 9.2.

The CT Scan of his abdomen revealed inflammation around the sigmoid colon with free fluid and air.

"Perforated colon," I explained to Mickey, "which will need surgery today. Most likely the cause is diverticulitis, but it could also be a tumor. We'll probably need to do a temporary colostomy, also."

"Whatever you need to do, Dr. Gelber, just make the pain better," he answered.

Funny thing about peritonitis; nobody that truly has generalized peritonitis ever says, "I don't think I want any surgery."

Mickey was wheeled into OR 10 about an hour later. A generous midline incision was made, and upon entering the peritoneal cavity, the surgical team was greeted by the foul odor of stool and pus which began to well up into the wound.

Ah, the sweet aroma of festering stool. A fine way to start my weekend.

"Suction, cultures, more suction," I called out as what seemed to be gallons of fetid, infected fluid were evacuated from his abdomen. There were thin adhesions between the loops of dilated small bowel that were broken with light finger dissection. This annoying small bowel kept trying to insinuate itself between me and the source of Mickey's woes. The inflammation led me deeper and deeper into the lower abdomen and upper pelvis until the culprit was isolated: a perforation in the colon at the rectosigmoid junction.

The small bowel was packed out of the way as I prepared to attack the evil villain who had fouled poor Mickey. The attachments of the left colon were divided to help me approach the area of perforation. As I carefully dissected, the small bowel decided it should try to help, and broke through the barrier of lap pads that I had vainly constructed to keep these intestines out of my way. I packed the small bowel out of the way again, this time using a wet towel instead of mere lap pads.

Now stay away.

I next did my best to identify the ureter and I was pretty sure I saw it as I gingerly searched beneath inflamed layers of fat and fluid.

My hands, then forearms, elbows, and almost my shoulders, disappeared into the depths of Mickey's abdomen as I did my best to dissect below the area of perforation.

Maybe I should have someone tie a rope around my waist so I don't get lost in this pelvis.

"There's a mass here," I announced to no one in particular as I managed to bring the diseased segment of bowel out of the pelvis.

At this point the resection proceeded quickly. The proximal colon was divided with a stapler, I managed to get a stapler below the area of perforation, and the bowel was divided and stapled closed. The mesentery, which contains the blood vessels, was divided with the usual clamp, clamp, cut, and tie of most bowel resections, and the rectosigmoid colon was removed and thrown on the back table to be examined later.

I checked Mickey's abdomen for bleeding, looked at the ureter again, and then washed out his abdomen with bucket after bucket of warm saline solution. Once I was satisfied that Mickey was clean, I examined the resected specimen.

It was about 20 centimeters long. About five centimeters from the distal end there was a hole about one centimeter in diameter. There was a hard mass just distal to this hole. I opened up the bowel and saw the tumor: ugly, ulcerated, almost filling the lumen.

"Not good for Mickey," I concluded. "Maybe all the stool in the belly killed any cancer cells that may have escaped."

Time to get on with the surgery.

"Three O Prolene," I requested. These blue Prolene sutures are used to tag the end of the rectum, making it easier to find should I came back in the future to reverse the colostomy Mickey was about to receive.

A colostomy is where the colon is brought out to the skin surface. Stool then passes into a bag, rather than its normal passage through the rectum and into the toilet. The bag is necessary because there is no sphincter muscle to control when and where the stool will pass.

Mickey stayed on a ventilator overnight. His recovery was remarkably uncomplicated, considering how sick he should have been. He left the hospital nine days after his surgery.

One week later he rolled into my office, smiling, feeling quite well.

"I feel great, Dr. G," he reported. "No pain, everything's working."

"That's great, Mickey. You look good," I answered as I took out his staples, perused his colostomy stoma, and palpated his rotund belly.

"When can I get rid of this bag?" he asked.

"Well, you need to heal a bit more and I think you'll need chemotherapy. The pathology report says there was cancer in two of your lymph nodes and the colon was perforated. We'll get you an appointment with Dr.

H to get his opinion about chemotherapy. After you're done with chemo, and assuming everything else is OK, we can schedule surgery to reverse the colostomy. I'll see you again in about a month."

And I sent him on his way.

Should be about six months until I have to tackle that belly again.

Wrong.

It was about 5 weeks later that Mickey's wife called my office and reported that Mickey was bleeding from his colostomy, mostly dark blood, but sometimes bright red. As an afterthought she added that he was having intermittent drainage from the midline wound through a tiny, pinhole opening.

"Bring him in," I responded.

An hour later, the massive form of Mickey, along with his diminutive wife, graced Exam Room Three.

"So, tell me what the problem is, Mickey," I began.

"Just take a look," he answered and he pulled up his shirt.

His colostomy bag was full of thin dark, bloody fluid. The skin was retracted, although he had done a good job of keeping his appliance in place. Adjacent to the colostomy his midline wound had a gauze dressing which was stained with yellow brown fluid.

"You're right, you are definitely bleeding. When did this start?" I asked.

"Two days ago. I'm not having any pain, Oh, and the colostomy doesn't stick out any more. It's been quite a chore getting the bag to stay."

"Well, I think you need to be back in the hospital; I'll get the GI doc to check out your colon to figure out why you're bleeding."

Please be something simple. I'm not ready to attack Mickey, his 400 pounds and his bowels so soon.

As he stood up to leave I immediately figured out the problem. Mickey's big belly hung down about eight inches below his belt line. Following his belly was his colostomy stoma, except his poor colon was tethered by its blood supply, causing it to pull on the skin. The stoma retracted under the skin while the blood vessels were stretched.

The final result was a portion of colon, which was both congested and ischemic, leading to the dark bloody drainage. The retracted stoma allowed the stool to collect beneath the skin level and form the sinus tract that was draining through his wound.

I shared my thoughts with Mickey and his wife, and tried to formulate a plan to correct the problem, something simple, I hoped.

Alas, it was to be everything but simple.

Once he was safely ensconced on the surgical floor at the hospital, Mickey stayed mostly in bed and the bleeding abated. My friendly neighborhood Gastroenterologist was consulted and colonoscopy scheduled.

I sat at Mickey's bedside and presented my plan to him and his wife.

"It's a little earlier than I'd like, but the simplest way to fix this problem is to reverse your colostomy," I explained.

They were both in agreement, his colonoscopy checked out OK, and surgery was scheduled for the following day, Friday.

It was noon when Mickey was rolled into OR 5. He scooted from stretcher to table like a lithe teenager, and in short order, the operation began.

The midline incision was made and the peritoneal cavity entered in the upper abdomen, above the area of his previous surgery and, I hoped, any adhesions.

Maybe this won't be too bad.

As if to punish me for having such thoughts, I ran into the proverbial wall, or, in this particular case, net of adhesions. Omentum plastered to colon which was wrapped around small bowel which filled the pelvis. No blue sutures to tell me where the closed-off stump of colon was hiding, but also, no cancer.

Minutes rolled into hours as I inched my way around bowels, omentum, and adhesions, finally spying one of my Prolene sutures after more than three hours of chiseling away.

I'm supposed to be doing a gallbladder in 10 minutes.

"Could you please call 'elsewhere hospital' and let them know I'm late. I may be there by four or four-thirty," I requested of my kind circulating nurse.

"Maybe doing this surgery earlier than planned was a bad idea," I remarked out loud to no one in particular.

"Looks like we're almost there," my assistant commented as more blue suture popped into view.

Sure enough the blue sutures which would lead me to the closed off stump of rectum now loomed large in front of me. A final snip freed the last loop of small bowel, which was then examined from beginning to end and safely packed away from Mickey's lower abdomen.

I now stared at a long tunnel that was Mickey's pelvis. Down in the depths was the object of my intentions: a stump of rectum which I hoped would accommodate the EEA stapler.

The proximal colon was dissected free from the abdominal wall and the big moment arrived.

The EEA stapler is a clever device which fires two rows of staples while cutting out two donuts of tissue between the circular staple lines. This leaves an opening between the two organs that have been stapled together. I find it most useful for constructing anastomoses at the ends of the GI tract, those involving esophagus or rectum.

This stapling device has a detachable part called the anvil which goes into one end of the colon, usually the proximal portion. An opening is made and the anvil is passed through this opening, which has had a "purse-string" suture placed, that is tied around the anvil, closing the colon wall around it.

I'll get one shot at this; it better work.

Mickey's bottom had already been prepped and I began the process of passing the stapler. First, the anus was stretched with a series of lubricated metal dilators up to a size adequate to allow passage of the stapling device. After the device has been inserted, it is guided to the proximal end of the closed-off rectum. The stapler was then opened and a spike appeared which pierced the closed-off rectum and then connected to the anvil. The stapler was tightened and fired, and then withdrawn.

The big moment arrived as the stapler was opened and the excised tissue "donuts" removed. In Mickey's case, the donuts looked complete, but very thin on one side. I next checked the anastomosis to see if it was airtight. I filled Mickey's pelvis with water so that the colorectal anastomosis was completely submerged. Next, I instilled air into the rectum and watched for bubbles. If the colon inflates, but there are no bubbles released, then the anastomosis is airtight. Bubbles percolating through the water mean there is a hole somewhere.

Much to my disappointment, a large number of bubbles appeared.

Now what? Do it again? You had one shot and you blew it.

Maybe do another colostomy? But what about his big belly? Problems, problems, always problems. Only skinny people should be allowed to get sick. At least we should get paid by the pound.

"We'll need to do a transverse colostomy," I announced to the OR crew.

I decided that creating a loop colostomy in the upper abdomen would minimize the pendulous abdomen issue while allowing my newly constructed coloproctostomy (colorectal anastomosis) the time to heal.

The new stoma was constructed with my usual workmanlike efficiency and Mickey was closed up. I had spent five and a half hours in Mickey's belly, battling large and small bowel, scar tissue and fat. As I pulled off my gloves, I felt a tightness in my knee, a common occurrence after long surgeries which command my singular attention for a long period of time.

Over the years I've discovered that cases like this require I concentrate on the surgery to the extent that I forget to move or change position, block out much of what is happening around me, be it my cellphone or music which may be playing, or the beeps and chimes coming from anesthesia's machines. The patient increasingly becomes my only focus as I become oblivious even to the pain that grows in my knee.

I wish I could say that every patient requires such intense concentration, but that wouldn't be true. Most surgeries are straightforward and, thank God, uncomplicated, such that this level of concentration is not necessary. If every case was like Mickey, I don't think I would still be practicing surgery.

Mickey recovered uneventfully. Three months later I checked his colon and found that the anastomosis in his pelvis had completely healed. He underwent an uncomplicated reversal of the transverse loop colostomy. I felt fortunate that I could stay out of his big abdomen and avoid further skirmishes with his bowel.

He remains cancer-free to this day.

9 ½ WEEKS

I met Alice almost by accident. Sunday morning rounds were nearly completed when I passed Dr. T in the hallway. We exchanged pleasantries and then walked on in opposite directions. But, seemingly as an afterthought, he called out.

"Do you think you can go by and see a patient for me? Her name is Alice. She's in Room 402. She's in the hospital with constipation and she's pretty distended. I plan a colonoscopy tomorrow, but maybe just give her a quick look. She had a CT that just showed constipation."

"Sure," I replied, "I'm going in that direction anyway."

Alice was petite, weighing in at 98 pounds, and she certainly was distended, almost like she was about to deliver twins. She was 46 years old, had always had "bowel trouble," had previous back surgery, and was on chronic pain medication, taking Percocet several times a day. She had not had previous abdominal surgery.

"Does your abdomen hurt?" I began.

"All over, but the Dilaudid helps," she replied.

"When did the pain start?"

"About three weeks ago, but it got worse three days ago."

"When's the last time you had a bowel movement?"

"Nine weeks before I came into the hospital."

I had to stop for a moment to completely absorb this statement.

I think this is a record.

"Did you say 'nine weeks'?" I asked again.

"Yes, nine weeks."

"...and you've been here three days, so it's been nine and half weeks since you had a BM? Is that unusual for you?"

"Normally I go every three or four days. I did start to panic after a week, but I didn't know what to do."

"Are you able to pass gas?"

"I'm not sure."

"Let me check your abdomen."

She was extremely distended and had diffuse tenderness, and some signs of peritonitis, particularly tenderness to light percussion on the right side of her abdomen.

"I'm going to look at your CAT Scan and then I'll be back."

So much for getting rounds done at a reasonable time.

The CT Scan done the day before revealed just what one would expect in patient who had been constipated for nine and half weeks. The colon was dilated, filled with stool, but not much air. The cecum, the first part measured 10 centimeters, approaching the diameter where blowout becomes a concern. The dilated colon stopped in the mid-sigmoid colon, which is just above the rectum. There was no definite tumor or mass, but there was a definite transition point from dilated to collapsed colon.

I checked her labs next. Her white blood cell count had been slightly elevated at 12,000 the day before, but today it had jumped up to 35,000. Her bicarbonate level was 14, which is low, normal being around 25. Low Bicarbonate suggests metabolic acidosis, a sign of severe metabolic derangement and sepsis.

Taking everything together, there was no question. She needed surgery. She either had perforated her colon or she had dead or dying colon. Either way, it was a life-threatening surgical emergency.

Of course, Sunday is not the best day to get anything done quickly. There were a series of Orthopedic cases scheduled already.

"I need to do this lady soon," I explained to the crew.

"It looks like you're in luck. Dr. R just cancelled his last two cases and we are finishing up with him now," the OR nurse reported.

"Good."

I explained my findings and concerns to Alice and her family, put her orders in the computer, and waited for the OR crew.

Maybe just a colostomy will suffice. But, it would be better to eliminate the cause of the obstruction. Quick and simple will be best for her.

After about 25 minutes, Alice was wheeled into OR Room 10 and was asleep a few minutes later.

A midline incision through the taut abdominal wall brought me into her abdomen which was filled with a few hundred cc's of slightly cloudy, yellowish fluid. I could see that the sigmoid colon was massively dilated, but it was not gangrenous. There was a faint, pungent odor.

Looks like I should be able to remove the offending portion of colon.

I could see where the colon transitioned to normal caliber just above the pelvis. I began to mobilize the colon by dividing the peritoneal attachments that tethered the sigmoid and left colon.

"Feels like there's a hard mass in the colon causing the obstruction," I observed out loud to no one in particular, my assistant nodding her head.

I should be able to get this colon free and then...

Before I could finish this thought the dam burst open and I was suddenly up to my elbows in thick, liquid stool.

"Shit..." Literally.

"Suction, lap, more laps, more suction."

The suction became plugged with stool. I squeezed the colon closed with my hand and it fell apart. Like The Blob from the 1950's or the river of slime from Ghostbusters, liquid stool took over.

"I need an intestinal clamp, something atraumatic," I said loudly.

The circulator scurried out of the room and came back with the GI instruments. In the meantime I had managed to isolate the source, rather the sources, of the river of stool and began to get at least a semblance of control.

The evil culprit then chose to rears its ugly head.

"There's a big rock of poop causing the obstruction," I noted.

Indeed, this "fecaloma" had completely blocked the sigmoid colon and eroded into the wall of the bowel, setting a trap for me as I mobilized the colon. As soon as the colon was free, it exploded, releasing its noxious contents. The resulting inundation left poop everywhere, on every loop of bowel, and filled the pelvis.

With the proper intestinal clamp in hand, I stemmed the flow and went on with the resection. I had to make two passes with the GIA to divide the dilated bowel while there was no difficulty dividing the distal colon, stapling it closed with the RL60 stapler.

Home free.

I finished resecting the sigmoid colon and examined it on a separate table.

This colon is as strong as soggy Kleenex.

"Uh, Dr. Gelber, I think there's a problem here."

"What…?"

Liquid stool was filling up the abdomen again.

I hurried back to the cesspool which was Alice's open belly and valiantly struggled to stem the flow again. The staples had not held the friable colon together. Once again, we went to work, sponging and suctioning until I could see enough to mobilize the colon away from its usual position on the left side of the abdomen, find the hole, and carefully put a clamp across it.

This time it held, at least enough to allow me to get my bearings and assess the situation in a calmer, more orderly manner. I made a closer inspection of the remaining bowel.

The right side of the colon didn't look very good either. Muscle fibers in the cecum were split under the tension caused by massive dilation; the ascending colon had patches of frank gangrene, as did the splenic flexure.

It all needs to come out.

Back to work. I began by dividing the attachments to the cecum and was then able to free the hepatic flexure with minimal fuss, and the remainder of the colon followed until everything had been mobilized. I zipped through the mesentery with the Ligasure, and before long the colon was resting in a large basin on the back table. At this point we all changed gowns and gloves and tried to banish the fetid, pungent odor from our

276 | *Amazing Days, Endless Nights*

nostrils. Even with benzoin (a fragrant compound often used in surgery) on our masks and repeated washing of hands, I knew that the fine aroma of stool and dead bowel would linger with me for the rest of the day.

This nasty beast has been far too much trouble. Time to finish this case.

We spent the next 20 minutes washing, washing, and more washing. Liter upon liter of warm saline was poured, sprayed, percolated, and pumped into every nook and cranny of her abdomen. We squirted irrigation fluid into the pelvis, above the liver, around the spleen, and between every loop of bowel until the fluid came out as clean as it went in.

Finally, I brought the end of the small bowel out to the abdominal wall to be matured as an ileostomy, took one more look around her belly, and closed her up.

Ensconced safely in the ICU, I washed my hands one more time, wrote orders, dictated the op note, and last of all, told her family the sordid tale of her surgery.

I called Alice's attending physician and consulted one of the Pulmonary docs, checked on Alice one more time, and finally left the hospital for the day.

Alice was kept on the ventilator. She was very slow to wake up from anesthesia and her blood pressure hovered in the 80's, occasionally dipping into the 70's. A massive volume of IV fluid and support with Levophed and Vasopressin were necessary to maintain an acceptable blood pressure. These two medications help maintain vascular tone, which helps maintain blood pressure in patients with septic shock. Her kidneys started to shut down, but timely adjustment of her fluids and medications by a Renal consultant turned this around.

The following day she looked a little better. She was more awake, had good urine output, but still required pressor support with Levophed and Vasopressin. She continued to smolder along over the next 48 hours, neither improving nor deteriorating.

I became a little concerned about her abdomen at this time as it became more distended and the ileostomy stoma looked dark purple instead of pink. Her lactic acid level rose to a very high 14, a sign of worsening acidosis, which indicated seriously poor perfusion of something and worsening sepsis. Although she maintained adequate blood pressure and kidney function, it became clear that something was amiss or amuck or afoul.

Alice was taken back to surgery.

The previous wound was opened and a couple of liters of clear fluid was drained.

That explains the abdominal distention.

In the lower abdomen there was some cloudy, foul-smelling fluid. As I gently freed up the small bowel and delivered it out of the abdomen, I discovered the new source of Alice's woes. The distal small bowel was dead, not completely, but patches had frank gangrene. I resected about 25 centimeters of terminal ileum and redid her ileostomy.

She also had a portion of abdominal wall that was dying and this also was excised. I put her back together as well as I could and delivered her to the ICU, hoping for the best.

The next 24 hours brought hope as she required less support with the pressors. However, she didn't wake up.

The following day came with new events that proved to be too much. She began to have cardiac arrhythmias, frequent Premature Ventricular Contractions (PVC's), and runs of atrial flutter and ventricular tachycardia. A

Cardiology consultant added his words of wisdom to the already exhaustive list of consultants.

"Acute MI," he said with a solemn expression on his face. "Ejection fraction is only 30%," he said shaking his head.

She's not going to make it.

Alice continued along for a couple of more days, but she didn't wake up, her kidney function gradually declined and her family wisely withdrew support, allowing her to pass away.

I wish I could report that timely surgery had rescued Alice. I don't know how many similar patients I've treated over the years; how many times I've told families, "We've eliminated the source of infection; the perforation, the blockage, the gangrene, the abscess; now it's time to heal."

Very often it's this healing phase which proves to be too much. Organ systems that have suffered the supreme shock of serious systemic infection are unable to recover and gradually shut down. The initial sepsis leads to what is called multi-organ system dysfunction, which progresses to multi-organ failure, which often leads to death.

After I finish operations such as Alice's, I've learned not to say: "Alice (or Andy or Mabel or anyone) will be better now."

I've learned that the human body often does not suffer lightly intrusions by combinations of bile, blood, GI contents, or urine mixed with microorganisms which thrive in such an environment. The body does its best to fight such invasions and often is successful. But sometimes, as all the body's warriors are mobilized and the battle is fought, the first wave of invaders may be defeated and the war looks like it will be won. However, sometimes the fight is too much, the strain is overwhelming, and the body dies.

And nine and a half week's worth of poop is more than most of us could handle.

REFLECTIONS

I began my medical career with those first moments in a lecture hall in Rochester, New York, September 1980. It wasn't long before I learned what ignorance meant. I progressed from this uninformed obliviousness through an explosion of knowledge, then comprehension, followed by a sense of understanding, which put me on the path towards skill and expertise.

Medical school led to residency where for five years I lived, breathed, dined, and slept surgery. I left residency with a sense of accomplishment and invincibility, believing that I could tackle any illness or injury. Years of practice, battling the worst diseases and injuries, replaced invincibility with humility. Finally, I settled on wisdom which comes with experience and occasional luck.

I've learned that the human being is a remarkable organism, demonstrating incredible resilience, displaying amazing powers of healing, often with a little help from health care professionals, and sometimes in spite of a doctor's best intentions. In the name of "medical treatment" spleens, pancreas's, kidneys, lungs, large parts of the gastrointestinal tract, brain, or liver may be removed, altered, or replaced while the body just shrugs its shoulders and goes on.

I've been in the practice of surgery for over 25 years. After so many years it would be expected that I would have perfected the craft. The only consistency has been inconsistency. No two patients, no two diseases, are ever exactly alike. This gallbladder is distended, that one is contracted, another is filled with sand-like stones, the next one with a single stone the size of a tennis ball. My years of practice have taught me to be careful and vigilant, to plan for and anticipate the worst, and to be grateful when disaster doesn't materialize and the outcome is good.

One thing which often leaves me pleasantly surprised is the gratitude my patients express, even when the outcome is far from optimal. Jack was one such patient. I had operated on him for carcinoma of the esophagus, discovering at surgery that the tumor was inoperable. All I could offer was some palliation, which in his case meant placing a gastrostomy tube so he could be fed. My office arranged for him to be seen by one of the medical oncologists, but he only survived a few months. Years later I crossed paths with his daughter. She greeted me and recounted how grateful Jack had been for all I had done. I didn't think I had done much, but her words touched me.

Our patients look for caring, for the sense that they are more than a piece of meat on a conveyor belt. A timely phone call, a word about their work or hobbies, even a pat on the shoulder which says, "I'm here for you," especially when there is little more to offer, is often the only thing which is remembered.

And, such tiny gestures may be enough.

MY SURGERY

It started about three and a half years ago: an episode of pain in my abdomen.

Not terrible pain, but a gnawing pain in my upper abdomen, coupled with a queasy feeling.

Probably just my GERD acting up.

I took my Prilosec and an antacid and went on my way.

The pain, however, stayed with me.

All day. And the next day. And the next.

This is annoying. It must be more than reflux. Maybe it's my gallbladder?

One would think that I would have thought of gallbladder disease first. I see patients with gallstones, dysfunctional gallbladders, biliary dyskinesia, and every other manifestation of biliary tract disease almost every day.

"Do you think you can do a quick sono on my gallbladder?" I asked Dr. L., a Radiologist friend. "I've been having epigastric pain for four days and I think it might be my gallbladder. That is, if you're not too busy and the ultrasound is available."

"Sure," he answered. "No doubt about it," he remarked a few minutes later. "Those are gallstones. You should get an official ultrasound if you are going to have anything done."

"Agreed," I answered as I went on my way, still with pain, but at least with the knowledge of what was causing the problem.

The next day the pain was gone. I thought about having surgery at that time, but the pain stayed away and I didn't think about it again until about five months ago.

The pain eventually came back, but different than before.

It's just my reflux. I'll go back on my Prilosec.

This pain was a little sharper than the previous, but only lasted about 20 minutes . . . at first.

The days went by and the pain lasted longer and longer, but still wasn't terribly severe. It was always in my epigastrium, and started lasting about an hour, occurring almost always in the morning. And, it got better if I ate, particularly a large meal.

Definitely atypical for gallbladder.

Pain from gallstones typically is worse after eating and often occurs at night. Pain in the morning, relieved by food, was more consistent with peptic ulcer disease.

Except, I'd had an Upper GI endoscopy only about a month before which did not reveal any ulcer.

Still, it was just an annoyance. And, I did have gallstones.

There was a change for the worse about two months ago. The pain I had was sharper, just to the right of the midline in the epigastrium and it persisted for about three hours. Then, it moved to my back for an hour before vanishing completely.

RUQ abdominal pain, lasting for hours, radiating to the back? No question. This is my gallbladder.

Still, I considered it an annoyance rather than something dire, something mandating immediate intervention. I occasionally took two Tylenol which helped, but otherwise went about my daily business.

Pain, however, can wear you down. Particularly when it occurs every day and lasts for hours.

A daily cycle began.

I awoke each morning feeling well. After about an hour the pain would start in my upper abdomen, always in the middle. It would intensify for about an hour. By the time lunch rolled around it would start to diminish and disappeared by early evening.

Every day.

You need to be a good patient.

I scheduled myself for an ultrasound of my gallbladder which confirmed a gallbladder packed full of stones. Then I went to see my partner, gave him the whole story, and scheduled my surgery.

I guess there's no way I can operate on myself? I'll just have to trust my partner.

We scheduled the surgery for a Friday about 10 days hence. The abdominal pain continued its daily pattern unabated. Some days the pain was sharper and lasted for 4-5 hours. It eventually moved to my back and then dissipated. Unlike so many of my patients who say the pain occurs at night, mine almost always started in the morning and disappeared completely by dinner time.

Three days before surgery, the pain was less, merely a mild gnawing ache which only lasted a couple of hours. Two days before surgery, I only felt a slight queasiness without real pain.

Maybe I don't really need this surgery.

But, the day before surgery the real pain returned.

I guess it's time.

The morning of surgery I did my usual thing: got up a little after 5:00, fed the bird, fed the dogs, fed everybody but myself.

My wife and I parked the car at 6:25 and went into Bayshore Hospital's Day Surgery.

"This way, Dr. Gelber, we've got the VIP suite ready," one of the nurses chimed.

"Room 15?" I answered. "Nothing very VIP about it."

Back in the old Day Surgery unit there was Room 22. It was larger and had its own bathroom. Now the only difference between Room 15 and the other rooms is that it is separated from the other rooms by a hallway. I suppose it does afford a little more privacy.

I donned my hospital gown and my red, no-skid socks, and lay down on the stretcher to wait.

It wasn't very long before two pre-op nurses descended. One asked the usual questions: medical history, allergies, previous surgery, was I wanted by the FBI; you know, routine.

The other started my IV. I pointed out my prominent "intern vein" which is at my right wrist and she started the IV like the pro she was.

There was another short wait until the anesthesiologist made an appearance. Unlike some other VIP's, I did not choose any particular anesthesiologist.

They all strike me as having equivalent levels of skill and I trust my patients with all of them.

Dr. M arrived and had me sign his consent. He didn't give me a lot of explanation, rightly assuming that I was well versed in the anesthesia routine.

Dinah and JR, who would be circulating and scrubbing the case, stopped in to say hello, asked if I had any questions or concerns, and then left to make sure the room was ready.

Finally, the star of this endeavor, the surgeon, Dr. L., arrived, 10 minutes early, a record for him.

He smiled, introduced himself to Laura, and said the surgery would take about an hour.

Finally time to start.

Dr. M made another appearance. He plugged an infusion of morphine into my IV, watched as the steady drip…drip…drip began, and left.

Dinah reappeared and we were off. I remember being wheeled down the hall and the doors to the OR Room, #8 I believe, opening, and that was it.

I can only imagine being asked to move from stretcher to table. I don't remember any of it. I suspect Dr. M said I might feel a little sting as the Propofol was injected, but I don't know for sure. There certainly was a time out, maybe a joke or two at my expense, and the ensuing surgery.

The next thing I do remember is being asked to breathe in the Recovery Room. Laura was sitting at the bedside. The PACU nurse asked if I was having any pain.

A little, certainly not excruciating. "Some," I answered.

A half-milligram of Dilaudid was pushed through the IV.

It worked. The little pain I had went away.

Once again I forgot to breathe, so that every so often I would hear, "Take a deep breath."

As a matter of fact, the accumulated Morphine and Dilaudid worked very well.

I couldn't stand up, couldn't pee, couldn't do much of anything for about four hours.

Finally, the narcotic effects started to wear off. With help, I made it to the bathroom, emptied my bladder, and was deemed fit to go home, about six hours after the surgery had finished.

Of course, I still felt the effects of anesthesia and narcotics. I drank a little water and went to bed. Winston, one our dogs, a Miniature Schnauzer/Pomeranian mix, made it his personal responsibility to oversee my recovery. He jumped on the bed, sniffed me all over, made sure I was breathing, then lay down beside me.

No doubt he's concerned about me, rather he's concerned that if anything happens to me he won't get fed.

After a couple of hours I took my first pain pill, an Ultracet which is relatively mild.

After seeing how I reacted to Morphine and Dilaudid, Dr. L rightly decided that 7.5 mg of hydrocodone might be too much for my delicate system and added the prescription for Ultracet.

The entire recovery was uneventful. I was able to eat without any problem. I took only two Ultracets. And I was back to work on Monday.

I looked at the photos from the surgery. The gallbladder didn't look inflamed; my liver looked normal.

"You had a lot of little stones," Dr. L. reported.

Makes sense, goes along with the pain I was having. Probably passed a little stone every day.

All in all it was, as best as I can tell, a boring operation. Perfectly mundane and boring. Which is the way surgery should be.

This cholecystectomy was my third experience with general anesthesia.

First was a fractured fibula which required a closed reduction in seventh grade. Then shoulder surgery after my second year of medical school.

Undergoing surgery, besides the benefit of eliminating the annoying gallbladder pain, should help me empathize with my patients. I now can say to my patients that I know what you are experiencing, even if I never

had to take anything stronger than Tylenol for my gallbladder pain.

Same story after this surgery, except for two Ultracet.

And, it does underscore the truth that every patient,
every illness, is unique.

We are all individuals and deserve to have our health
care tailored to our personal needs. This fact is not evidence based and doesn't fit into any standard protocol.

It does, however, lead to happy patients and good
care.

DEAR SON,

Congratulations on being accepted and starting medical school.

Your long hours of hard work have paid off. We are so very proud of you. Your journey into the world of medicine will be fascinating, tumultuous, inspiring, tiring, educational, interesting, and frustrating, and so much more.

I'm sure you are not looking for any advice from your old father, but I will give it to you any way.

Read, learn, read some more, and then jump in and do as much as you can.

It is true that learning about the rhomboids and intercostals is tedious, but every muscle, blood vessel, and nerve in the human body has a purpose.

It is fascinating to see how different cells come together to make tissue and how a combination of tissues becomes an organ. The way these organs interact to make a human and how infirmity can circumvent normal functions sums up all there is to learn about the art of medicine.

As you study, you will be surprised at how individuals, your patients, live and function while battling disease and pain.

Later, as you travel through your medical career, you will be amazed at the resiliency of these patients.

They may suffer through cancer, heart disease, trauma, deadly infections, and so much more, and still get up each morning and face each day with hope and probably a shrug of their shoulders.

As you progress from basic science to clinical medicine, try to remember that the "chest pain" you are asked to evaluate at 3:00 a.m. is a person; one who has a home and family and life apart from his illness.

Remember that your patients are going to be frightened at the prospect of suffering through a serious, maybe life threatening ailment. Your job is to ease their suffering and their fears. Learn to use your medical skills to be caring, informative, reassuring, and compassionate.

But, for now, absorb as much information as you can from your lectures, books, and labs. Later, learn from your patients. Learn to talk to them, to ask the right questions, but mostly learn to listen, because 98% of the time they will tell you what is wrong.

And, when the time comes that you have to tell someone that the end is imminent, that the best that can be done is to make them comfortable, do so with compassion.

If you find yourself feeling overwhelmed, worrying that you haven't done all you could have for one of your patients, take a step back. Reflect on all that you have done; review in your mind, your thoughts and actions.

The vast majority of the time you will have followed the proper course. I know that I have done this hundreds of times as I stand at the bedside of a sick post-op patient or think about the day's events as I lie in bed trying to sleep.

Sometimes, hindsight will tell you that a different treatment would have been better. These are educational moments which make you a better physician.

Finally, remember that there is a world away from medicine. Take the time to get away the day-to-day struggles and worries all doctors face.

Play your music, read for fun, spend time with friends (extra points for not discussing medicine).

Welcome to medicine. Enjoy yourself, don't worry, and have fun.

Love,
Dad

ABOUT THE AUTHOR

D r. David Gelber has been practicing surgery in the Houston, Texas region for nearly thirty years. He is a Fellow of the American College of Surgeons, a Diplomate of the American Board of Surgery and is currently Chairman of the Department of Surgery at Bayshore Medical Center in Pasadena, Texas.

He has been named one of America's Top Docs by Castle Connolly on multiple occasions, was named one of Houston's Top Five Hundred Physicians by Houstonia magazine, and has won the Patient's Choice award.

His surgical skills range from removing simple lumps and bumps to performing complex cancer operations and managing severely injured trauma patients.

He has been married to Laura for over thirty years and has three grown children. His home is a menagerie which currently numbers five dogs, two cats, and two birds.

In addition to *Amazing Days, Endless Nights* he has written two additional books about surgery: *Behind the Mask* and *Under the Drapes*; the three comprise the *Mystique of Surgery* series.

In addition he has authored numerous works of fiction: *Future Hope ITP Book One, Joshua and Aaron ITP Book Two, Little Bit's Story, Minotaur Revisited, Night Clinic* and *Last Light.*

Dr. Gelber's blog is called Heard in the OR, a place where his essays with topics ranging from saving turtles to his unique Super Bowl predictions can be reviewed.

His website is http://www.davidgelber.com.

He can be contacted at david@ruffianpress.com.

BOOKS BY DAVID GELBER

Behind the Mask: The Mystique of Surgery

Under the Drapes: More Mystique of Surgery

Amazing Days, Endless Nights: Mystique of Surgery Three

Future Hope: ITP Book One

Joshua and Aaron: ITP Book Two

Little Bit's Story

Minotaur Revisited

Night Clinic

Last Light

CPSIA information can be obtained
at www.ICGtesting.com
Printed in the USA
FFHW011813250119
50224793-55229FF